# KID FOOD

# KID FOOD

THE CHALLENGE OF FEEDING
CHILDREN IN A
HIGHLY PROCESSED WORLD

BETTINA ELIAS SIEGEL

LIVINGSTON PUBLIC LIBRARY
10 Robert Harp Drive
Livingston, NJ 07039

OXFORD
UNIVERSITY PRESS

# OXFORD

UNIVERSITY PRESS

Oxford University Press is a department of the University of Oxford.
It furthers the University's objective of excellence in research, scholarship,
and education by publishing worldwide. Oxford is a registered trade mark of
Oxford University Press in the UK and certain other countries.

Published in the United States of America by Oxford University Press
198 Madison Avenue, New York, NY 10016, United States of America.

© Bettina Elias Siegel 2019

All rights reserved. No part of this publication may be reproduced,
stored in a retrieval system, or transmitted, in any form or by any means,
without the prior permission in writing of Oxford University Press,
or as expressly permitted by law, by license, or under terms agreed with
the appropriate reproduction rights organization. Inquiries concerning
reproduction outside the scope of the above should be sent to the
Rights Department, Oxford University Press, at the address above.

You must not circulate this work in any other form
and you must impose this same condition on any acquirer.

Library of Congress Cataloging-in-Publication Data
Names: Siegel, Bettina Elias, author.
Title: Kid food : the challenge of feeding children in a highly processed
world / Bettina Elias Siegel.
Description: New York, NY : Oxford University Press, [2020] | Includes
bibliographical references and index.
Identifiers: LCCN 2019001198 | ISBN 9780190862121 (hardcover : alk. paper)
Subjects: LCSH: Children—Nutrition. | Children—Health and hygiene.
Classification: LCC RJ206 .S57 2020 | DDC 613.2083—dc23 LC record available at
https://lccn.loc.gov/2019001198

1 3 5 7 9 8 6 4 2
Printed by Sheridan Books, Inc.
United States of America

*for Dana*

# CONTENTS

# NOTE: A WORD ABOUT "HIGHLY PROCESSED" FOOD

Throughout this book, I use the term "highly processed" to describe certain foods and beverages. But what does it mean?

In its PR materials, the food industry tells us that "processing" is "any deliberate change in a food that occurs before it's available for us to eat," whether it's "as simple as freezing or drying food to preserve nutrients and freshness, or as complex as formulating a frozen meal with the right balance of nutrients and ingredients." By defining the term so broadly, the industry can then offer all kinds of reassuring messages, like: "most of the food we eat is processed" and "food processing began about 2 million years ago" (referring, I suppose, to fire-roasted wooly mammoth?). The industry and its supporters also like to remind us—frequently—that even frozen fruit, bagged salad greens, and baby carrots are all "processed" foods.

Those statements are literally true, and it's also true that modern food processing provides all of us with an unprecedented degree of food safety and convenience. We shouldn't discount the importance of those achievements, nor should we romanticize our preindustrial past, when food-borne illness was far more common and when preparing and preserving food was an exhausting, full-time endeavor—especially for women.

At the same time, though, food's most basic purpose is to nourish the body and foster health. If it causes harm, something's clearly gone off the rails—and I think we all know the problem doesn't lie with frozen fruit and baby carrots.

Because the industry's definition of "processed food" includes both the pear that's been sliced and dried *and* the unfortunate pear that winds up in a box of Betty Crocker Blastin' Berry Hot Colors Fruit Roll-Ups (ingredients: Corn Syrup, Dried Corn Syrup, Pear Purée Concentrate, Palm Oil, Citric Acid, Sodium Citrate, Fruit Pectin, Monoglycerides, Malic Acid, Dextrose, Ascorbic Acid, Acetylated Monodiglycerides, Natural Flavor, and Color [Red 40, Yellows 5 & 6, Blue 1]), I would argue that the term has ceased to have any real meaning. So for the purpose of our discussion here, I've turned instead to a classification system called "NOVA," which was first put forth in 2009 by Dr. Carlos Monteiro, an expert in nutrition and public health at the University of São Paulo in Brazil.

The NOVA system assigns all foods and beverages to four categories, the last of which is "ultra-processed." (You can find a description of the other three categories in the endnotes.) Ultra-processed foods and drinks are industrially produced, contain at least five ingredients (but usually many more), and—in addition to salt, sugar, and/or fat—typically contain industrial additives not commonly found in our kitchens. Sometimes these additives are themselves highly processed, like hydrogenated oils and soy protein isolate. NOVA's examples of ultra-processed foods include mass-produced: sweet and savory snacks; ice cream, candy, and cookies; breakfast cereals; energy bars; pre-made pizza and pasta dishes; poultry and fish nuggets or sticks; burgers; hot dogs; and packaged soups, noodles, and desserts.

When I first read the NOVA definition, though, I was actually inclined to reject it because it seemed to reflect a certain distasteful food snobbery. Like, why is a carton of mass-produced vanilla ice cream considered an "ultra-processed" food (with all of that term's negative connotations) while a batch of homemade vanilla ice cream is merely "processed?" After all, a few industrial additives likely make little difference to our bodies, and in the case of some mass-produced vanilla ice creams, such as Häagen-Dazs's, the product's ingredient listing reads like a recipe we might use in our own homes: cream, skim milk, sugar, egg yolks, and vanilla.

But when I read further, I learned that the NOVA system builds into its definition of ultra-processed food a number of external factors that clearly *do* make a difference to our bodies, by pushing us toward overconsumption of less healthy food while luring us away from healthier, whole foods. Specifically, in discussing ultra-processed food, the NOVA team includes this statement:

> The main purpose of industrial ultra-processing is to create products that are ready to eat, to drink or to heat, liable to replace both unprocessed or minimally processed foods that are naturally ready to consume, such as fruits and nuts, milk and water, and freshly prepared drinks, dishes, desserts, and meals. Common attributes of ultra-processed products are hyper-palatability, sophisticated and attractive packaging, multimedia and other aggressive marketing to children and adolescents, health claims, high profitability, and branding and ownership by transnational corporations.

In other words, what makes the mass-produced vanilla ice cream problematic is the very ease with which we can buy it cheaply and consume it in great quantity, and the degree to which we're encouraged to do so by a constant barrage of sophisticated and aggressive marketing. None of that is true of homemade ice cream, which takes time and planning to make—precisely why so few people ever undertake the project, even when they actually have an ice cream maker languishing in their kitchen cabinets. Most mass-produced foods are also hyper-palatable, as the NOVA team notes, meaning their flavor and texture have been carefully calibrated to make them extremely pleasurable to eat—so pleasurable that some experts believe they're actually addictive, or at least potentially so.

In this way, the NOVA definition of ultra-processed food squares nicely with one of food writer Michael Pollan's most oft-repeated *Food Rules:* "Eat all the junk food you want as long as you cook it yourself."

I realize there are still some gray areas in NOVA's definition. Would hand-churned vanilla ice cream from a family-owned shop still be merely "processed?" What if the shop used artificial additives but never engaged in marketing? Some people have criticized the NOVA system for these inconsistencies, along with its obvious anti-corporate bias, and I've cited a few of these critiques in the endnotes. But even with this admitted fuzziness on the margins, I still think the NOVA definition gives most of us

NOTE

a pretty clear mental picture of the foods and drinks in question. At any rate, it's exponentially more precise than the self-serving definition offered by the food industry.

I use "highly processed" in this book as a synonym for NOVA's "ultra-processed" category just because I prefer it stylistically. But in light of the correlation between a diet high in ultra-processed foods and beverages and a host of serious health concerns, I sometimes just refer to these products as "unhealthy"—or, where it feels especially warranted, as "junk food."

NOTE

# KID FOOD

# INTRODUCTION

When it comes to feeding their kids, most parents start out with the best of intentions: They simply want to raise healthy eaters. But even before our children climb down from the high chair, it can feel like junk food is coming at them from every direction.

We take our toddlers grocery shopping, and though they can't yet read, they easily recognize the cartoon characters beckoning from boxes of the least healthy, sugary cereals. At restaurants, a smiling server hands our preschoolers a kids' menu offering the same six entrées you see everywhere—as though some federal law mandates that children under ten eat nothing but foods that are batter-fried and beige. And later, when they're old enough to go to school, our kids may encounter snacks like Rice Krispies Treats and Cheetos Fantastix in their cafeteria, PTA fund-raisers selling donuts or pizza, or a teacher doling out candy rewards.

Then there are days when every adult who crosses your child's path seems determined to offer him "just one treat." The bank teller hands him a lollipop—a sweet tradition you remember fondly from your own child-hood. But then he's offered a second lollipop at the drycleaners, a third when he goes for his haircut, followed by a Popsicle after gymnastics class. The music teacher happens to choose that day to bring in a box of donut holes. Even the pediatrician's office may offer candy to ease the stress of a check-up. But only the most uptight food-cop parent would object to "just one" of anything, so in each instance you squelch your objections—while also mentally canceling that ice cream outing you were going to propose later as a fun surprise.

We do our best to act as nutritional gatekeepers, but it's an uphill battle all the way. A decision to let your tween use Snapchat opens the door to "fun" filters from companies like McDonald's and Taco Bell, which essentially turn your kids' photos into junk food ads. A quick dash into Office Depot for school supplies turns into a pitched battle over buying candy from the kid-eye-level racks in the checkout aisle. (Because of course your *office supply* store needs to sell *candy*.) It's an endless game of Whack-a-Mole, and eventually, just out of sheer exhaustion, parents find themselves making dietary compromises they never would have dreamed of only a few years before.

Compounding this junk food deluge is the fact that some kids can be stubbornly resistant to eating healthier foods. So even when you do manage to get a home-cooked dinner on the table (an achievement that really ought to earn today's time-strapped parents a gold medal), it might well go untouched. And that's when you find yourself reaching for the highly processed grocery products every kid loves—the boxed mac and cheese, the sugary yogurt tubes, the chicken nuggets—while silently praying that the nutrient claims plastered all over their labels ("contains calcium!" "made with whole grain!") actually mean something, because: that's it, you're *done*, and everyone just needs to get *fed*.

Although my kids are older now, I totally understand what today's parents of young children are up against. I've even become known as an outspoken advocate on these issues, although that's something I never saw coming. I'm not a dietitian, pediatrician, or child-feeding expert, and I don't even play one on TV. Instead, I'm a former lawyer—and one who used to work for Big Food, at that. But when I try to pinpoint exactly how I wound up on this unexpected life path, I always come back to a brief conversation I had in 2010 about, of all things, animal crackers.

I was a fledgling freelance magazine writer back then, having left the legal profession a decade earlier when we'd moved from New York City to Houston. Our son and daughter (then eight and ten) attended our local elementary school in the Houston Independent School District (HISD), but although I was a stay-at-home mom, I wasn't the kind of parent who was eager to get involved in school or district affairs.

Then one evening my friend Donna called and asked if I'd be interested in joining a new HISD committee that was forming to gather parents' input about its school food menus. My first thought was that the district certainly could use the help. A typical lunch in 2010 might have featured a fried or cheesy entrée like "Texas Frito Pie" or chicken-fried steak fingers, often served with carb-heavy sides like mashed potatoes, sugary canned fruit, and a brownie, and kids usually washed it all down with carton of chocolate milk. If our district were trying to set students on a path toward poor health, it could hardly have done better.

I preferred to send our kids to school with a home-packed lunch, so I told Donna that since we weren't participating in the meal program, I wasn't sure I had a legitimate place on this new committee. But when Donna pointed out that we'd both gladly forgo the tedium of daily lunchbox packing if the school food improved, I couldn't disagree. So a few weeks later, the two of us walked into a conference room in HISD's administrative headquarters and joined other parents for an introductory presentation about our district's nutrition services department.

One of the first things I learned from this "School Food 101" PowerPoint was that more than 80 percent of Houston's public school students live close enough to the poverty line that they qualify for federally subsidized free or reduced-price school meals. In other words, for the majority of my fellow HISD parents, the food in the cafeteria wasn't an option to be weighed against a home-packed lunch but instead a daily necessity. I was ashamed I hadn't known so many families depended on school food, and suddenly the idea of improving it took on new urgency.

The second eye-opening fact I learned was this: After overhead, we were told, our district had about a dollar and change (per child, per meal) left over from its federal funding to pay for food. That shockingly low figure would certainly explain the subpar meals I'd been seeing in my kids' cafeteria, but I still couldn't quite wrap my head around it. Was there some fiscal mismanagement going on? Shifty accounting practices? Just what was being included in this mysterious "overhead" that was diverting funds from buying better food for our district's kids?

The last surprising moment came during a discussion of HISD's breakfasts, which are provided free of charge and eaten at kids' desks at the start of the school day. According to various studies, we were told, "in-class breakfast" is a proven way to get more hungry kids fed while reducing nurse's visits and discipline problems. But the food itself left a lot to be desired: shrink-wrapped, artificially flavored "maple" pancakes; glazed honey buns; snack packs of sugary cereal; and cartons of fluorescent blue Trix yogurt. I also learned that on four out of every five days, HISD students were required to take a package of animal crackers along with their meal.

This last detail was too odd for me to stay silent, so I raised my hand and asked, "Can you tell us why we're serving animal crackers almost every day at breakfast?" Without missing a beat, the district's dietitian replied, "Well, students are required to have a certain amount of iron every week, and the animal crackers provide it." Seeing my obvious confusion, she added, "You know, from the fortified white flour."

As I drove home from the meeting that morning, my mind was reeling—particularly about those animal crackers. It wasn't so much what the dietitian had said about iron and white flour, it was the utterly blithe tone in which she said it. To her, and apparently to the rest of our nutrition services department, giving kids sugary, white-flour cookies along with a sugary, highly processed breakfast was a perfectly fine way to fulfill children's *iron* needs. And somehow the federal regulations under which these people were operating made this an entirely acceptable choice. It was baffling.

Maybe because of my legal background, or maybe because I'm a nerd at heart, I wanted to dig deeper for answers. As soon as I got home, I searched Amazon for a primer about the National School Lunch Program and saw that one had been published only a few weeks before. And reading this book—*Free for All: Fixing School Food in America*, by sociologist Janet Poppendieck—was a revelation. It not only answered all of my questions about school food, it addressed many others I hadn't been knowledgeable enough to formulate.

After first outlining the school food program's origins as an anti-hunger initiative in the 1940s, Poppendieck explained how and why schools had abandoned scratch-cooking in favor of today's heat-and-eat fare. I learned why schools sell à la carte snacks like chips and ice cream, and I also discovered that HISD's shocking "one-dollar-for-food" figure was not only legitimate, it was actually true of almost every district around the country. And yes, by the time I finished the book, I even understood how we'd wound up with animal crackers for breakfast.

Meanwhile, parents at my children's school had learned at a PTA meeting that I was now a member of the district's new school food committee. As a result, there were days when I couldn't walk through the halls after drop-off without someone buttonholing me to complain about our school meals. But while I still shared these parents' concerns about HISD's subpar food, reading *Free for All* had put everything in a new light.

For example, while I didn't condone serving pepperoni pizza with mashed potatoes and brownies, *Free for All* had taught me that school meals (then) had no calorie maximum—a relic of the program's anti-hunger origins carried over into an era of childhood obesity. And although I still didn't approve of animal crackers at breakfast, I now understood that HISD was using the (now-obsolete) "nutrient standard" method to create its menus, which allowed districts to check off various nutrient boxes (like iron) without necessarily having to justify the bigger picture (cookies at breakfast). Most of all, I was now mindful of how very little money my district had to work with while trying to serve more than 250,000 school meals a day.

I knew few parents had the time or interest to investigate these issues on their own, though, and I was eager share what I was learning. I wanted to offer them a bigger picture of the problems driving unhealthy school meals, while also conveying my newfound empathy for the people serving them under enormous regulatory and budgetary constraints. But noisy school hallways aren't the best place to impart nuanced information, so I'd find myself nodding along with complaining parents while feeling a growing sense of frustration over all I wasn't able to say.

Around this same time, I also had growing concerns about our elementary school's overall food environment. My son's second grade teacher had rewarded him with M&M's for every correct math answer. Without asking parents' permission, the school gave students juice pouches and peppermint candy on standardized testing days in a bid to boost their scores. Seemingly every other week, my kids came home with icing-smeared faces, having just eaten another classmate's birthday cupcakes, while classroom parties tended to be veritable orgies of unhealthy food (one was actually called a "junk food party"!). And while I had no problem with my daughter's teacher using a system of "brownie points" to reward good behavior, did the points really have to be redeemable for actual brownies?

None of this would have bothered me very much if my kids weren't constantly offered junk food *outside* of school, too. My daughter's Saturday soccer practice meant "refueling" with Lay's potato chips and a Gatorade at 10 a.m. My son's daily snack at a half-day summer chess camp (because chess is so strenuous, kids can't make it to noon without one?) had included Kool-Aid Jammers, Nerds candy, Fritos corn chips, and Fla-Vor-Ice frozen ice pops. Even an outing to the supermarket meant a friendly employee handing my kids a large sugar cookie, a store tradition likely meant to keep children quiet while their parents shopped. (But of course, once that cookie had been waved in front of them, saying "no" would produce precisely the opposite result.)

And while we didn't keep a lot of highly processed food at home, I was dismayed at how well my kids knew these brands—and how much they wanted them. By preschool, both of them had been able to easily identify unhealthy snacks and cereals just from their packaging, and when we later let them watch popular kid shows on cable TV, their knowledge of these foods increased exponentially. I'd also made the mistake of letting my son become a regular player of "PopTropica," an online game touted to parents as an especially safe learning environment for children as young as six. Because I'd naively relied on that assurance of "safety," I only discovered much later that the game was littered with ads for Tootsie Pops, Apple Jacks, and Fruit Loops, and that it actually forced players to engage in brand-sponsored challenges, led by their cartoon mascots, before children were allowed move on to the next activity.

These brands' powerful influence on my kids became clear in the grocery store, where they often begged for products they'd seen advertised or at friends' houses. I hated having to be the "mean mom," always denying their requests for this or that unhealthy food, and sometimes out of sheer exhaustion I'd give in to at least one demand by the time we reached the checkout aisle. At the same time, I'd berate myself for caving on products I knew weren't good for them.

Once my children started encountering all of this unhealthy food in their daily lives, it also seemed as though healthier foods, like fruits and vegetables, were becoming an even harder sell. I cooked a family dinner almost every night, but when my kids resisted that meal, as they were increasingly doing, I'd often resort to surefire crowd-pleasers like Annie's mac and cheese, Amy's frozen pizza, and Bell & Evans chicken nuggets. Because those products all came from Whole Foods and were "clean label," I convinced myself that I was still feeding my children healthfully; in reality, I was only reinforcing their love of bready, fried, and cheesy flavors. And when we dined out and they were handed a children's menu invariably featuring these same types of foods, it only compounded the problem.

The surprising thing was, I'd never expected this particular aspect of parenting to be a challenge. Because of the way my own mother had raised me in the 1970s, I'd been certain that when I had children of my own someday, I'd know exactly how to feed them well.

I realize that sounds like I was weaned on tofu and kale, but in my earliest memories, my family's pantry was actually stocked with the best the processed food industry had to offer: Duncan Hines cake mixes, Hunt's pudding packs, and chewy Space Food Sticks—"the snacks taken into space by NASA astronauts!" as their ads told awestruck kids. We even had a now-discontinued miracle of modern food science called Jell-O 1-2-3, a brightly colored gelatin powder which, when combined with water, separated into a three-layered, multi-textured parfait. (How was that even possible?)

But I also grew up in the early 1970s—the Watergate era—when trust in big food companies and the federal agencies regulating them was at a low point. It didn't help that some widely used food additives, like the red dye in my favorite M&M's, had recently been banned for causing cancer in lab animals. Safety scares like those, along with alarming new reports about harmful pesticide residues in food, only further undermined Americans' confidence in the food supply. Suddenly the idea of "natural food" was moving beyond the hippie counterculture and gaining popular appeal.

My mom eventually tapped into this new zeitgeist, but the shift didn't start in her kitchen. Instead, it began in her flower garden, which was so lush and colorful that people often stopped in front of our house and took pictures of it. Troubled by what she was learning about chemical pesticides and fertilizers, my mom started to adopt organic gardening methods, like unleashing mail-order ladybugs on the aphids, putting out little saucers of beer for unwitting snails, and starting a towering compost heap out back. These new organic techniques paid off and her garden never looked better.

Then one day, when my mom was out weeding her flower beds, she had a disturbing epiphany. "I suddenly realized," she told me decades later, "that I was feeding my flowers so much better than I was feeding my own children."

My mom started to read books by progressive food advocates like Frances Moore Lappé and popular diet gurus like Adele Davis and Gaylord Hauser, and we soon became regular patrons of our town's only "health food" store, a cluttered little shop with a distinctly 1960s vibe and thickly scented with dried herbs, incense sticks, and stale vitamins. While my mom did her food shopping, I'd wander through the personal care aisles, intrigued and puzzled by those text-dense Dr. Bronner's soap labels ("Rise to the stars above and thrill!" "Arouse the very flames of life!") and sniffing at little tins of beeswax lip balm that looked like they'd been cooked up in some hippie's basement (they probably were).

These shopping excursions eventually transformed my family's pantry and eating habits. Gone were the cake mixes and pudding packs, replaced by canisters of brown rice and whole oats, boxes of rose-hip tea, and a stack of carob bars that were somehow supposed to take the place of our beloved Hershey's (prompting the question: who first had this idea, and had they ever tasted actual chocolate?). We bought a special plastic container to sprout alfalfa seeds and mung beans for our salads, and my mom started regularly baking her own oatmeal "cookies": dark brown disks, sweetened only with a touch of honey and blackstrap molasses, that no kid in their right mind would accept as a lunchroom trade for a Twinkie or a bag of Bugles. (On the plus side, they were so nutrient-dense from their brewer's yeast, flax seeds, and wheat germ, you could probably subsist on them indefinitely.)

This evolution from Jell-O 1-2-3 to mung bean sprouts was likely more gradual than I now recall, and we certainly continued to eat some processed foods throughout my childhood. All the same, though, I grew up with the definite sense that I was eating quite differently from my friends. It wasn't just that my classmates' sandwiches were on Wonder bread—so soft you could ball it up in your hand—while mine were on dry and dense whole wheat. It was that I was being taught that our food choices *mattered*, a lesson I absorbed from the home-cooked meals on our table every night and through frequent discussions about food with my mom.

So when my husband and I had our own two children, I was quite confident that I had a solid grounding in good nutrition. And while he and I were both adventurous eaters who loved exploring Houston's endless array of hole-in-the-wall ethnic restaurants, at home we typically ate healthy, scratch-cooked meals. With the two of us naturally modeling for our children both an enthusiastic openness to new flavors as well as good daily eating habits, how could we possibly go wrong?

With all of this swirling around in my head, I met my friend Jenny, a fellow writer, for lunch one day and tentatively said, "You know, I think I might start a blog about school lunch—but maybe also about kids and food generally?" Jenny gave me an assessing stare and then responded without hesitation, "You *have* to." And that was it. I came home, discovered the domain name "The Lunch Tray" was still available, set up a WordPress template and published my first post the following morning.

Nine years and almost 1,500 *Lunch Tray* blog posts later, my entire life has been turned upside down. Not only did the blog upend my budding career as a freelance magazine writer, it eventually pushed me so far outside my comfort zone that I now almost can't recognize the rather conflict-averse mom who sat in her pajamas that first morning, typing up her debut post at her kitchen table. These days, I'm known as an outspoken advocate on issues relating to children and food, and I've had some pretty remarkable experiences along the way, including:

+ waging three viral and successful online petition campaigns relating to school kids and food (including one regarding so-called pink slime in school meals), making me one of the most effective petitioners in Change.org's history,
+ being highlighted in a congresswoman's TED Talk on the effectiveness of grassroots food activism,
+ breaking a story about McDonald's that was picked up by *Today* and the front page of the *Washington Post*, creating unwelcome publicity that forced the company to scrap a deceptive marketing program for kids, and

+ being named one of the nation's "20 Most Influential Moms" by *Family Circle* magazine.

I've also been able to reach more people with my writing than I could ever have dreamed, including through an opinion piece about school food for the *New York Times*, as well as a front page *Times* news story about "lunch shaming"—the practice of stigmatizing kids in the school cafeteria when they have overdue lunch accounts. The lunch shaming article went viral on social media, which led other national and local news outlets to publish and air their own stories on the topic. Thanks to that intense media spotlight and the public outrage it aroused, a number of states have since passed legislation seeking to ban lunch shaming.

As my expertise and visibility grew, I also became a sounding board for parents around the country—in my blog's comments section, at speaking engagements, and via the angst-ridden emails I received from readers on a regular basis. And what I learned from all these interactions is that my own concerns were hardly unique. Other parents clearly shared my sense that very little in our society's food system and food culture supports parents in their desire to raise healthy kids.

And yet, in responding to my readers' questions and pleas for help, I often felt uncomfortable—almost fraudulent. These parents saw me as an expert and understandably hoped to walk away from our exchanges with a solution to their problems. I willingly shared my best advice—how to try to improve school food in their district, for example, or how to get junk food out of their child's classroom—but I was always painfully aware that many of their concerns were rooted in much larger societal problems, ones that can't be solved solely through individual action.

Like so many of these parents, I'd had a vague sense that I was swimming upstream in trying to feed my kids healthfully. But after almost a decade of writing and advocating on these topics, I now understand clearly why that current feels so strong. And while many of the forces pushing kids toward unhealthy food affect adults, too, it's really our children who are in the crosshairs.

Children's bodies are vulnerable and rapidly growing, which means their diet can have significant and lasting consequences for their long-term health. The foods eaten in childhood can also shape taste preferences for a lifetime, yet our society's particular notion of "kid food" is especially unhealthy. Young children's brains are immature, which means they absorb junk food advertising uncritically, while older children are strongly influenced by social media, an especially powerful marketing channel the industry eagerly exploits. And unlike the rest of us, young children are dependent on caregivers and institutions for the food they eat. Lacking an adult's greater knowledge and critical thinking, they simply take for granted the food environment in which they live, drawing implicit but often harmful nutritional lessons based on whatever food they're offered by the trusted adults in their lives.

So my first goal for this book is to offer you a closer look at our children's junk-food-saturated days, teasing apart the various reasons why they encounter so much unhealthy food in so many different contexts. I'll explore the role of "picky eating" in driving children's poor diets, and how the processed food industry exploits parents' mealtime worries and guilt to promote its products. I'll explain why so many school meals still look like junk food, even after recent federal reforms. And I'll also point out all the ways we adults quite knowingly exploit children's love of junk food for ends having nothing to do with nourishment, like controlling their behavior, covering shortfalls in school budgets, reaping corporate profits, and even securing their love.

I next want to empower you, as best I can, to push back against the forces that drive your kids toward unhealthy eating. How can individual parents help improve their children's daily food environment, from school classrooms to sports leagues? How much power do we have in pushing food and beverage companies to do better? And for those of us who want to drive more systematic change through individual and grassroots advocacy, how can we make our voices heard?

At the same time, though, I want to be transparent about the limitations of individual efforts in some of these areas, asking you to also consider fundamental shifts in national policy that could make a real difference for America's kids. And for those of you who recoil at the idea of governmental intervention to solve some of these problems, I'll offer my best case for reconsidering that view.

I should admit up front, though, that I take on all of these topics with some trepidation. From my years of blogging and speaking about these issues, I've learned that just talking about our children's food environment—let alone how we might improve it—takes more than a little courage and a very thick skin. People who've found my concerns about children's health overstated, or the solutions I endorse overly intrusive, have called me everything from a "Food Nazi" to an "angry mommy"—as well as a few less-family-friendly epithets, sometimes with bonus anti-Semitism or misogyny thrown in for good measure. I've also been scolded by readers who think I'm not health-conscious *enough*, as when I once dared to explore the nutritional benefits of sugar-sweetened chocolate milk for kids, or when I've expressed more concern over getting fruits and vegetables on school lunch trays than whether those foods are organically grown.

None of that backlash should come as a surprise; our attitudes about food tend to be deeply personal, and discussions of food policy can be politically divisive. But I've also found that emotions run especially high in discussions about feeding children in particular. Most adults who work with kids—teachers, daycare operators, coaches—genuinely care about children's welfare, so when they're accused of harming them through their food choices, they can understandably feel angry or defensive. That's all the more true in heavily regulated contexts like the federal school meal program, where a school nutrition director's best intentions can be stymied by reams of red tape and insufficient funding.

And when it comes to moms (dads, too—though moms still do most of the grocery shopping and cooking in this country), nourishing a young child is a fundamental, even primal, act of parenting that can trigger all kinds of insecurities: Is my child eating enough? Too much? Why does my friend's kid love garlic-fried squid while mine eats only bananas and buttered noodles? It doesn't help that how we feed our children has become yet one more battlefield in the endless Mommy Wars. If you rely too heavily on highly processed foods, other mothers may accuse you of negligence, "poisoning" your child, or even child abuse. Swing too far in the other direction and you might be called a gullible alarmist, a control freak, or—my personal favorite—a "sancti-mommy."

These sensitivities all provide dry tinder for conflict over food issues, but I would argue that the flame is the food industry's influence on our elected officials, which in turn shapes our public conversations about food. Politicians on both sides of the aisle accept Big Food's lobbying dollars, to be sure, but the industry has predictably found the most receptive ear among pro-business, anti-regulation conservatives. And these politicians typically use charged, partisan language to protect their benefactors' interests: efforts to curb even the worst of the industry's abuses are "nanny state" intrusions on our "freedom," while public health advocates are finger-wagging "food police" bent on "telling the rest of us how to eat." This flag-waving, "pro-freedom" messaging is then amplified in the news and on social media by armies of paid public relations professionals, many of whom operate covertly behind front groups that hide their financial ties to the industry.

Due in large part to this unholy melding of partisan politics and the food industry's financial interests, anyone who cares about improving our food environment risks being mocked as an elitist foodie, while a carefree embrace of unhealthy food is a sign of being a "real" American. Why else do politicians of all political stripes—even the famously ascetic Barack Obama—feel the need to chow down on junk food while the cameras are rolling? It doesn't seem to matter that some of these politicians might hold very different views about food in private. Case in point: in 2011, former New Jersey governor Chris Christie openly applauded Michelle Obama's school food reform efforts, poignantly citing his own lifelong struggle with obesity. Five years later, he sarcastically mocked those same efforts to court conservative Republicans in the 2016 presidential primary.

For all of these reasons, pushing for change—whether asking one teacher to stop passing out candy or advocating for federal reforms in Congress—can be quite intimidating. Just daring to question the status quo can invite stinging criticism, whether from fellow parents or (if you're ruffling bigger feathers) PR firms, politicians, and powerful corporations. It's much easier for all of us to just keep our heads down and muddle through, struggling to raise our own kids in a society that seems permanently and hopelessly saturated with junk food.

I also understand that not everyone is a fiery activist out to change the world. Most parents are challenged enough just making sure everyone is dressed and out the door on time, with completed homework and signed field trip forms safely in their backpacks, and that something vaguely resembling "dinner" shows up on the table at the end of the day.

That's why I want help you navigate your child's food environment *as it is*, whether that's sharing the latest expert advice on picky eating, helping you decode confusing nutrition claims on product packaging, or pointing you to resources that can help even the busiest families eat together.

At the same time, though, I want to offer you a more hopeful vision of what that food environment *could be*—for your child and for all the children whose parents are too marginalized or disempowered to advocate on their behalf. Because polls show that the majority of American parents do support policies that would undoubtedly improve kids' health, from better school food to fewer junk food ads targeting their children. Yet very few of us actually vote on issues like these, or even think to hold our politicians accountable for them.

What would our children's world look like if we actually did?

# 1

# KID FOOD
# HOW DID WE GET HERE?

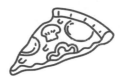

*Once given the choice of French fries, pizza, pasta, and chicken fingers,
my kids don't usually want to eat anything off the regular menu.*

~ MOM OF TWO, WASHINGTON, DC

A few years ago, before I'd ever thought about writing a book, I once randomly declared to my husband, "You know, sometimes I wish I could go back in time, and instead of studying law, I'd study history. And you know what my thesis would be about? Children's menus!" At Martin's blank stare, I helpfully added, "I mean, don't you ever wonder about that? Like, when they first started and why they're all the same now, and whether we always fed kids this way in restaurants?" [Another blank stare, now slightly tinged with pity.]

*Whatever.* Once I knew I was writing this book, I couldn't wait to dig into all the existing scholarship to finally get some answers. If I could just nail down what Americans used to consider "kid food," I thought, maybe

I'd better understand when and how it all went so horribly wrong. But after several days of coming up short in my research, I started to wonder if Martin's blank stare had been justified after all. Maybe I really was all alone in my (totally *not* weird!) obsession with the children's menu.

Undeterred, I did what any self-styled historian would do: I dove into the primary sources myself (in my case, online menu archives) to try to figure out when kids' menus first appeared and what they offered. But in the midst of this research, I was so taken with the retro illustrations on a particular 1930s-era railway children's menu that I posted it on Twitter. And in one of those lovely moments of social media serendipity, that menu was spotted by someone who wasn't even one of my Twitter followers, who then referred me to the blogger at *The American Menu*. He, in turn, referred me to Andrew P. Haley, a cultural historian at the University of Southern Mississippi. And Haley, it turned out, had written *the* definitive paper on the role of children in the American restaurant industry.

Talking to Haley on the phone was like finding my kid-food history soulmate (sorry, Martin!). And while his research focused less on my particular interest—the food served to kids—and more on why kids were being served in the first place, Haley's paper introduced me to a central figure in the history of children's menus: Ethel Maude Colson.

To say that Colson invented the modern-day children's menu would be an overstatement, but not by much. In 1920, she wrote an editorial in the trade journal *The American Restaurant*, with a title that asked the industry for the first time: "Why not children's luncheon?" And the ideas she suggested—a special menu just for kids, including "a cheap little toy or some similarly ... child-delighting feature"—were clearly new. When the journal's editor enthusiastically endorsed the concept in the same issue, he noted that "to the best of our knowledge," it "has never been done anywhere."

Haley didn't have any more information on Colson, so I assumed she worked in the restaurant industry. But I later discovered that wasn't the case at all. Instead, she was a writer—and an incredibly prolific one at that. She penned fiction, poetry, books on the analysis and writing of poetry, plays, radio scripts, literary criticism, and even song lyrics. She also worked at one time or another at every major newspaper in Chicago, both as a reporter and as an editor.

On top of all that, in 1927 Colson became one of the few female lecturers at Northwestern University, teaching journalism to young women. She also wrote a book that same year about opportunities in journalism for aspiring female writers (honestly, did this woman ever sleep?) in which she stressed that "the 'woman's angle' is the woman writer's tool." In other words, according to Colson, a female journalist's best hope for success in a male-dominated field was to focus her reporting primarily on "women's interests, ways and work."

And when seen in that light, it actually makes perfect sense that Colson, despite having no connection to the restaurant industry—or even children of her own—wound up writing about children's menus. Because for a certain well-heeled subset of women in the 1920s, the lack of a kids' menu was in fact a matter of growing interest and concern.

To understand why, you need to put yourself in the shoes of a mom in the early twentieth century. Food science had just begun to explore the role of "vitamines" and other nutrients in preventing malnutrition and disease, and these findings had been widely shared with the public during World War I as part of a federal nutrition education campaign. Meanwhile, women who'd been barred from careers in food science had carved out their own turf—the new field of home economics—and they, too, were offering a lot of expert guidance on how to feed one's family.

So if you were a mom of reasonable means and general awareness in the 1920s, you were suddenly on the receiving end of a lot of imposingly "scientific" nutrition advice which you ignored at your child's peril. All of this clearly influenced Colson, too, who opened her editorial by noting that "[t]he question of food for children is interesting the American public now as never before," and that "the right kind of food is too often not provided for the growing child, the citizen of the future."

So just what was the "right kind of food" for kids? Apparently, it wasn't anything found on a regular menu for adults. "The ordinary child, confronted by the glorious possibilities of a restaurant menu, is apt to order unwisely," Colson warned, or beg his mother for "foolish, forbidden dainties." (I laughed at Colson's quaint term for unhealthy treats, especially since today's restaurant executives would gladly ply kids with unlimited McForbidden Dainties to get them in the door.)

But Colson also understood that moms in the 1920s faced a new problem. Children were now occupying a more central role in family life because parents were having fewer children and giving each one more time and attention. So it was becoming more common for kids to accompany their parents on various outings, including weekend shopping excursions "in town" with their mothers. And as parents of any era can attest, nothing spoils a shopping outing like a hungry, cranky child.

So even before Colson's editorial appeared, a handful of department stores and ladies' tea rooms had already spotted this need and were offering special meals for children. But most regular restaurateurs had no interest in serving kids, whom they regarded as noisy irritants certain to drive away adult diners. (Haley's paper is full of the industry's amusingly unvarnished views about children, aka those "tyrants" in "short jackets and pinafores.") In fact, the hospitality industry generally did everything it could to keep kids away, including sometimes requiring children to eat with their nannies at different times of day, or even in entirely separate dining rooms in the case of hotels and resorts. They also typically refused to give parents any kind of price break when they dared to dine out with their kids.

But by the time Colson wrote her editorial, the industry was already beginning to soften. The change didn't reflect any newfound fondness for the tiny tyrants, though; instead, it was a response to Prohibition. The 18th Amendment, which banned the sale of alcohol, had been ratified three months before Colson's editorial appeared. But thanks to the temperance movement, the majority of states had already been dry for years and restaurant owners were seriously feeling the pinch. According to Haley, they lost not only revenue from alcohol sales but also the enticingly illicit, adults-only atmosphere that alcohol had provided. Meanwhile, a lot of bars were hastily reinventing themselves as restaurants, which meant competition for diners was growing fierce.

So the industry was already getting comfortable with the idea of serving families, but it took women—female customers, female restaurateurs, and commentators like Colson—to promote the idea of special printed menus and meals specifically for children. Alice Foote MacDougall, one of New York City's most successful restaurateurs at the time, said she first offered a children's menu in 1927 after a mom complained about the lack of "suitable dishes" for her young son. The menu proved so popular that MacDougall encouraged the rest of her industry to follow suit, later telling a trade reporter that "mothers who now dread having the children downtown for luncheon, because they find it so difficult to control their orders and appetites, will soon prove the financial feasibility of the idea."

As for the food served, Colson envisioned a menu that followed the era's child-feeding advice, which meant a lot of dairy (milk was considered the "best and most important food" for kids) and simple, bland foods—or, what another trade journal later called "the greaseless diet so beneficial to children." Specifically, she suggested serving "daintily cooked cereals, perhaps, good soups, creamed fish or chicken, simple salads and desserts, milk, plain or flavored as in chocolate or cocoa, brown bread, plain ice cream and so on." And this is pretty much what most restaurants offered, not just in the 1920s but right into the 1950s (and even later, at some particularly antiquated restaurants): dairy-based dishes like creamed chicken on toast or creamed spinach, along with beverages like milk, buttermilk, and cocoa; eggs served poached, coddled, or in jelly omelets; vegetable- or cream-based soups; chicken sandwiches; and simple broiled meats like chicken or lamb chops.

Most striking, though, was the emphasis on vegetables. A significant number of children's menus actually offered vegetables as an *entrée* (parents: can you *imagine?*). These came in the form of the vaguely named "vegetable plate" or "vegetable luncheon," which meant either a selection of various cooked vegetables or a meatless entrée accompanied by vegetables. And the side dishes on children's menus were also almost always vegetables, such as buttered peas, carrots, and asparagus.

This isn't to say that restaurants didn't try to please kids' palates. But even the sweet treats on most children's menus seemed to reflect an underlying concern for nutrition. Desserts were usually fruit-based, like stewed pears, applesauce, or "prune whip" (which sounds gross but was apparently beloved in its day), or milk-based, such as puddings, custards, and vanilla ice cream.

Restaurants were also willing to amuse kids by presenting their food in fun and novel ways. For example, by 1929 the Chicago department store Marshall Fields was serving an astonishing 1,200 children every Saturday and another three hundred daily during the week in its six tea rooms, and among its popular children's entrées were chicken croquettes "formed in a tin" and "served in the shape of a chicken." (Have we just identified *the very first chicken nugget* served in America?)* Another popular item was—prepare yourselves—"sweetbread croquettes made to look like an eye, with a dot in the center." I can't decide what's more surprising: that kids in the 1920s were happily tucking into cow thymus glands, or that they were thought to be even more appealing when made to resemble an eyeball.

But children's menus weren't just helpful to moms while dining out; they were also seen as a way to boost kids' overall acceptance of healthier foods. A 1929 trade journal article said moms were going to Marshall Fields specifically "to cultivate their [children's] taste for certain dishes despised at home." Kids who hated milk apparently found it had "different appeal" when "served in miniature glasses with nursery figures engraved on them," and "the same goes for spinach and other health-building vegetables that youngsters do not especially relish." A 1930 article on other restaurants' children's menus similarly noted, "Many of the [children's] dishes are selected for variety of color as well as flavor, for no eye is so much attracted by color as that of the child's. Thus, beets having one hue, spinach another, carrots a third and peas a fourth, the child can be intrigued by the rainbow effect on its plate if they are deftly arranged."

Just let that sink in for a second. In the old days, a children's menu was seen as a tool to help kids overcome picky eating. Could anything be *less* true of today's kids' menus, which seem specifically designed to reinforce children's worst eating habits?

Take the sixteen items on the current children's menu at the restaurant chain Chili's, all but one of which draw from the standard, unhealthy universe of pizza, cheeseburgers, corn dogs, and their ilk. The Red Robin kids' menu offers kids "bottomless" servings of soda and milkshakes. And while today's children share the same "attraction to color" as kids in the 1930s, the restaurant chain Friendly's satisfies it not with a "vegetable rainbow" but a candy-filled pancake ("Color outside the lines! Better yet,

---

* Credit for the chicken nugget is given alternately to McDonald's, which introduced the McNugget in 1981, or to a Cornell University professor who proposed a frozen, breaded "chicken stick" in 1963. But I'm going with Marshall Fields and its little chicken-shaped croquettes.

color your way to delicious Tie-Dyed Pancakes with M&M's for break-fast!") and a bright turquoise children's drink called "Sharks in the Water"—described as "gummy sharks [that] circle in a pool of blue raspberry Sprite with a side of shark bait (red syrup)."

Keep in mind that restaurant owners were no less profit-driven in the 1920s and 30s than they are today. Colson championed the children's menu to make women's lives easier, but she also chided restaurant owners for being "slow to realize the financial opportunity" in front of them, promising they'd make "good money" in feeding kids. And once they did follow her advice, restaurateurs realized that a nagging child is a powerful marketing tool. As one trade reporter wrote in 1930, "[T]he youngster is . . . to be cultivated and encouraged" because "[m]any a mother has been persuaded to eat in a certain restaurant merely because that establishment's management has been especially attentive to Johnny."

But even though restaurants were more than happy to make a buck off little Johnny, they still didn't try to entice him with the sort of menu he'd likely choose for himself—swapping out the creamed spinach for more ice cream and pudding. Instead, ever mindful of the era's newly nutrition-conscious moms, the industry mainly stuck to non-food treats to lure kids in, like menus printed with nursery rhymes, games, and songs, or illustrated bibs that could be taken home.

Of course, since Colson's day, the entire American way of eating has undergone a shift that could fairly be described as seismic. We've seen the dramatic rise of agribusiness and the processed and fast food industries, along with a related decline in home cooking—a decline so steep that we now spend more on food prepared outside the home than we do on groceries. Few Americans are eating very well anymore, kids or adults, so some might say it's pointless to lament a bygone era when children were happily eating "vegetable luncheon" followed by stewed pears.

Even so, it still feels like somewhere along the way, our society simply threw in the towel when it comes to looking out for kids' best dietary interests. Just as we currently let adults smoke and drink while restricting the sale of alcohol and tobacco to minors, children in Colson's day were (at least ideally) kept in a nutritional "cocoon" until they were old enough to make grown-up decisions about food. But today, we've reversed that paradigm. Even restaurants like Chili's and Friendly's offer salads and soups on their adult menus, but their kids' menus remain mostly a nutritional wasteland. It's as though we've all embraced the illogical notion that kids will wake up one day and suddenly start eating more healthfully, even though we seem determined to wean them on unhealthy "kid food."

What exactly is "kid food"? There's no precise definition, of course, but in 2018, I conducted online survey asking my readers and other social media followers what the term meant to them. About 350 people responded—mostly moms, but some dads and even a few grandparents also chimed in. And just one glance at their top answers, ranked here in descending order, tells you a lot about what American adults currently believe children will and won't eat:

- chicken nuggets
- Goldfish crackers
- pizza
- Cheerios
- hamburgers
- sugary cereal
- French fries
- mac and cheese
- juice boxes
- hot dogs and corn dogs
- "white" or "beige" food
- grilled cheese or quesadillas
- packaged "fruit" snacks
- noodles or pasta
- milk
- apple slices
- baby carrots

There's nothing particularly kid-centric about pizza, burgers, and fries, of course, and milk, carrots, and apples are certainly healthy. But taken as a whole, my readers' list is clearly dominated by foods that are relatively bland yet undeniably tasty, thanks to a heavy use of salt, sugar, refined grains, and fat. Many are also hand-held items that, in the words of one child feeding expert, kids can just "gum, squish, and swallow."

Another way of gauging our culture's conception of "kid food" is to simply stroll through the average American supermarket and look at the kinds of products aggressively pitched by food companies (to both parents and kids) as being especially "for children." It's a profitable marketing strategy that took off in the 1930s, when breakfast cereal manufacturers started putting cartoon mascots like Tony the Tiger and Snap, Crackle, and Pop on their boxes. By the 1950s and 60s, the cereal aisle was awash in sugary brands specifically marketed to children, but it wasn't until the mid-1990s to the early 2000s that "kid" versions of other kinds of foods began to proliferate in earnest.

Since then, breakfast cereal has lost its footing as the dominant "kid food" grocery category, with child-centric products now found in almost every aisle. That said, food manufacturers seem to particularly equate "children's" products with "super-sweet" products. In looking at market research showing all the new, kid-focused grocery items introduced since 2013, seven of the top eight product categories represented were sugary: candy, yogurt, juice, breakfast cereals, cereal bars, processed fruit products, and cookies. (The eighth and largest category was savory snacks, like crackers and chips.)

But if everything from yogurt to a frozen dinner can become "kid food" in the hands of the processed food industry, there does tend to be one unifying characteristic across all these product categories: the enticing promise of "fun." Whether through the use of appealing or unusual food shapes, colors that don't exist in nature, cartoon characters on their packaging, promotions involving giveaways or games, and/or the fact that kids can manipulate or play with the food before eating it, "kid food" products typically convey to children that they're in some way a form of *entertainment*. And from these "fun" products, as well as restaurant children's menus, kids are clearly absorbing some troubling messages about what "their" food is supposed to look like. When children were asked in a 2012 Canadian study what the term "kid food" meant to them, they most often mentioned "junk," "sugar," fun shapes, and unusual colors. "Adult food," on the other hand, meant unprocessed and generally healthy foods like fruits, vegetables, and meat.

My 2018 reader survey also asked parents where their kids were most likely to encounter unhealthy kid food (outside their own homes).

The resulting list would be funny if it weren't so sad—virtually no aspect of a child's day went unmentioned. In roughly weighted order, they listed:

+ their child's school
+ restaurant meals
+ school aftercare and daycare
+ team sports practices and games
+ other afterschool activities like club and scout meetings
+ religious school, church dinners, and other faith-based activities
+ play dates
+ summer day camp and sleep-away camp
+ time spent with grandparents and other relatives
+ and a few other miscellaneous contexts.

Or, as one disgruntled mom summed it up: "Everywhere we go outside of the house."

But even though our children are glutted with unhealthy "kid food" (including, at times, in our own kitchens), I think adults recognize on some level that we're selling kids short. Most of us are at least vaguely aware that there was once a time when families typically sat down to the same dinner, when special "children's" versions of various foods would have puzzled the average grocery shopper, and when no one had ever laid eyes on a fish-shaped cracker. (Today, an astonishing half of all American households with children reportedly buy Goldfish.)

But if we need any further proof that the human child actually *can* survive without mac and cheese, we only have to look to two scientific experiments in which a group of toddlers happily subsisted—for years— on nothing but whole foods like kidneys, lettuce, barley, and bone marrow. Really!

The studies in question took place in the late 1920s and 1930s and, as with the rise of children's menus, they were a response to that era's new theories about child nutrition. Specifically, pediatricians were now thinking about food in terms of its constituent nutrients, thanks to modern food science, and they also regarded children's digestion as particularly delicate. So they often strictly dictated the exact types and amounts of food mothers should offer their children, as well as the time of day when it should be offered. Not surprisingly, a lot of kids rebelled—so much so that according to one doctor writing in 1930, 50 to 90 percent of all pediatrician visits related to "anorexia," or a child's refusal to eat.

But not everyone agreed with this new feeding advice, and among the skeptics was a Chicago pediatrician named Clara Davis. Davis not only felt her colleagues were going overboard with their regimented approach, she also suspected that if kids were free to feed themselves, they might naturally choose all the right foods to meet their bodies' needs.

It was an intriguing theory but one that would be hard to prove, since it would necessarily require studying children away from any parental influence. So Davis came up with a study design that was, to put it bluntly, pretty wacky—and not a little unethical by today's standards. She persuaded impoverished widows and unmarried young mothers to turn their babies over to her as soon as they were weaned, to be raised by her and a nursing staff in an orphanage-like setting where Davis could completely control and observe the children's food intake. She also specifically sought out babies who'd never seen solid food—making them, in her words, "as yet untampered with" with regard to their "theories, tastes or habits with respect to food." In the end, Davis found fifteen such children, ranging in age from six to eleven months, and in some cases they remained in her study for as long as four and a half years.

Davis then drew up a list of thirty-three foods she believed would provide all the necessary "food elements" for human nutrition: fourteen different fruits and vegetables, plus orange juice; grains like oatmeal, barley, corn, and wheat; chicken, beef, lamb, and fish; organ meats like brains, liver, kidneys, and sweetbreads; bone marrow and bone jelly; and sea salt. These foods were to be served to children on a rotating basis, with a few items from each category offered at each meal. Davis also dictated that no two items could be combined, which meant her subjects were never exposed to common mixed foods such as bread or soup.

Instead, each individual food was prepared as simply as possible and served in its own separate dish (even the salt), and some foods were offered both raw and cooked (including, yes, raw beef, eggs, and bone marrow.) The only drinks offered were water, milk, and "sour milk," and after these items were laid out on a table, the child's nurse was instructed to "sit quietly, spoon in hand, and make no motion" until the child pointed to a given dish. They were also told not to "comment on what he took or did not take, point to or in any way attract his attention to any food, or refuse him any for which he had reached."

With these protocols in place, Davis quickly discovered that no two children ate alike, and that even on a day-to-day basis any given child's food choices were unpredictable. A toddler might demand a breakfast of orange juice, barley, and liver one morning, only to ask for apples, brains, and kidneys the next. Over time, Davis also noticed that many kids went through food jags—eating one particular food with ever-greater frequency "until astonishingly large amounts were taken" for a period of time. Ultimately, Davis came to believe that children possess an innate "body wisdom" drawing them to the nutrients they most need. Children who'd recently been sick, for example, reportedly ate more raw beef, carrots, and beets, while a baby who'd arrived at the orphanage with rickets quite willingly drank the cod liver oil included in his food selections— but only until he was healed.

In the end, Davis concluded (maybe a bit smugly) that "not one diet was the predominantly cereal and milk diet with smaller supplements of fruit, eggs and meat" that her fellow pediatricians said was essential for children. In fact, despite their complete failure to follow that dietary advice, Davis's toddlers were in excellent physical health, at least based on growth charts, blood tests, and X-rays. Davis described them as a "rollicking, rosy-cheeked group," while a doctor who'd visited her orphanage called them "the finest group of specimens . . . I have ever seen."

Davis published only one paper documenting her work, in 1928, and it focused on just three of her toddlers. The rest of what we know about her experiments comes from a series of speeches she delivered in the 1930s. But her work still strongly influenced the parenting experts of her day. In 1941, psychiatrist Leo Kanner wrote in his (excellently titled) book, *In Defense of Mothers: How to Bring Up Children in Spite of the More Zealous Psychologists*, that "every mother ought to be acquainted" with Davis's findings, which proved there was no need to "sacrifice peace, dignity and a child's comfortable relationship to his family on the altar of nutritional dogmatism," adding that "eating is not a major issue unless and until a major issue is made of eating." And when pediatrician Benjamin Spock published his landmark *Common Sense Book of Baby and Child Care* in 1945, he, too, cited Davis's experiments to reassure worried parents that they "can trust an unspoiled child's appetite." While not exactly what Davis set out to prove, her experiments also clearly show that children will eat all kinds of non–"kid friendly" foods, at least by modern American kid standards (again: *raw* bone marrow!). But what if processed foods like cookies and white bread—what Davis called "incomplete, altered, and sophisticated foods"—had been offered alongside the cabbage and kidneys? How would her toddlers have responded then?

To find out, Davis planned as her next experiment to raise children in the same setting, this time offering the healthy items on her list *and* less healthy processed foods. Did the human appetite have "innate fallibilities" that would always draw it to processed food, she wondered aloud in one of her speeches? Or do we humans have an innate desire to eat healthy food that's only "overruled" by processed food's external attributes, like its "novelty, cheapness, ease of procurement and preparation?"

Davis never conducted that follow-up study because the Great Depression scotched her funding. But today, it's as though all of our children are unwitting subjects in that exact experiment—and they prove on a daily basis just how "fallible" their appetite is whenever there's processed kid food on offer. Here are some relevant quotes from my reader survey:

+ "Ugh. Go to a soccer game and see the kids dive into the Rice Krispies Treats and ignore the fruit."
+ "My son will not touch a veggie if there is 'kid food' around."
+ "If there are chicken nuggets, nothing else gets eaten."
+ "Who wouldn't take a cupcake and Goldfish crackers over a salad?"

Yet because our children are conditioned to expect kid food in so many contexts, *not* offering it can come with a steep price. A summer camp director may worry that kids will write home to complain they're "starving" if she doesn't stock their unhealthy favorites in the mess hall. A manufacturer may fear a drop in sales if its children's products contain less palate-pleasing sugar, fat, and sodium than those of its competitors. And we know with certainty that restaurant executives are terrified of losing customers if they stray too far from unhealthy kid food on their children's menus.

How do we know the latter? Because in 2010, First Lady Michelle Obama asked the restaurant industry to do just that: to offer items on their kids' menus that "actually are healthy" and which would "help our children get into habits that will last them a lifetime." She made this request in a speech to the National Restaurant Association, and her goal was ambitious: instead of the usual corporate window-dressing, Obama asked restaurant executives for "a commitment to promote vegetables and fruits and whole grains on every part of every menu," and not "just one token healthy option."

The restaurant industry responded in 2011 with a program called "Kids LiveWell," touted as a "first-of-its-kind initiative" that "showcases the restaurant industry's commitment to offer healthful options for children." But if you read the fine print, you'll quickly see that this voluntary program requires of its members only the "token" commitment the First Lady had specifically criticized: restaurants can qualify for the Kids LiveWell designation by offering just *one* children's meal, along with one additional individual item, that meet certain caloric limits and which also include healthy foods like fruits, vegetables, whole grains, or lean protein.

As of this writing, 150 restaurant chains in 42,000 locations have joined the Kids LiveWell program. But because of the low bar for entry, the food offered to kids at these restaurants varies wildly. The Silver Diner chain embraced the challenge and swapped out the fries on its kids' menu for fresh strawberries, mixed vegetables, and steamed edamame. But many other chains have done only the bare minimum, which is why, if you squint, you'll find one lonely grilled chicken breast among the fifteen unhealthy children's entrées on that Chili's kids' menu I mentioned earlier. The weakness of the program also explains why Friendly's (with its "Tie-Dyed" M&M pancakes and "Sharks in the Water" candy-drink), and Red Robin (with its bottomless sodas and milkshakes) can also proudly tout their Kids LiveWell membership.

It's still good news that grilled chicken breasts and the like are available on at least some children's menus, and several major restaurant chains have also recently dropped sugary drinks as their default kids' beverage. But to use Ethel Colson's words, you do have to wonder how many kids willingly choose the grilled chicken when still confronted with so many other "unwise" but "glorious" options.

Meanwhile, because the ratio of healthy-to-unhealthy food on children's menus typically remains so skewed, when Harvard researchers checked in on Kids LiveWell chains three years after the program began, they still described their children's menus as "dismal" and basically unchanged in terms of overall calories, salt, and saturated fat. And a 2017 study found that even when chains listed healthier kids' options online, they often weren't offered at individual restaurants.

The whole notion of "kid food" is of course an artificial construct (today's mac and cheese is yesterday's "vegetable luncheon"), but our current unhealthy iteration, driven in large part by food industry marketing, is stubbornly self-perpetuating. Businesses and institutions that live or die by pleasing kids—restaurants, summer camps, school cafeterias—are understandably afraid to push too far ahead of consumer demand. So they cling instead to the lowest common denominator foods that few children will ever reject, while keeping any nutritional improvements safely at the margins. It's a surefire way to garner a little good PR without actually driving kids away.

One way to break America's unhealthy kid-food cycle, then, is to raise little consumers who will happily embrace—or even demand—healthier food. And in light of Clara Davis's barley-and-beet-eating toddlers, it doesn't seem like this should be such a tall order. But if babies come into this world with an innate openness to non-"kid friendly" foods, why do so many parents have children who steadfastly reject them?

# 2

# THE BEIGE AND THE BLAND

*Our daughter is a chicken nugget, pizza, waffle kid.*
*The Brown Food Diet, I like to call it.*
*It's an endless battle—and it's extremely hard to undo once it's done.*

~ DAD OF ONE, NORTH SCITUATE, RHODE ISLAND

There's no more confident parenting expert than the person without kids. Before our two children came on the scene, I knew I'd never use television as a babysitter or lose my cool over sibling squabbles (because my kids would coexist in perfect harmony, of course!), and I was also convinced that the whole idea of "picky eating" was a myth. If a friend complained that her toddler "wouldn't eat" vegetables, or would "only eat" buttered pasta, I'd nod along in sympathy while secretly thinking it was all just the product of bad parenting.

When I eventually did become a mom, I had no reason to revisit my judge-y views. Our daughter accepted new foods pretty willingly, so instead I had several lovely years in which to bask in the glow of my obviously superior parenting skills.

Then our second child came along.

Like his older sister, our son was at first happy to eat any puréed food, even strongly flavored vegetables. But almost as soon as he was old enough to pick up finger foods from his high chair tray, he started to show worrisome signs of pickiness. With ever-increasing frequency, any vegetable I offered went untouched, until one day in his third year he actually looked up quizzically from his lunch to inform me: "Mommy, I don't *eat* vegetables." The polite tone in which this news was delivered was hilarious—as though I'd missed an important intra-family memo and he was just kindly bringing me up to speed.

But I shouldn't have laughed, because it turned out this kid *meant* it. As in: even years later, he was still was resolutely avoiding all vegetables and sometimes also fruit, despite my haphazard application of every strategy I could think of—from trying hard to stay hands-off, to creating colorful sticker charts, to the "For the love of God, *just take just one bite!*" approach I'd resort to in moments of total despair.

That was just the beginning of my painful and well-deserved comeuppance about picky eating. As I shared with you in this book's introduction, once our kids were a little older, I started falling into the kid-food trap without really thinking about it. My husband's job back then meant frequent travel and long hours, so we couldn't always sit down to a shared family dinner. But as our kids started eating more highly processed food outside the house, they seemed less interested in whatever I'd cooked anyway. It became all too easy to serve a quickly prepared "kid" meal at 6 p.m., then enjoy an "adult" dinner with my husband after the kids were asleep.

In many ways, everyone was happier with this arrangement. Our children were getting more of the pasta and quesadillas they loved, and my husband and I were getting some rare adult conversation over a glass of wine. Maybe precisely because of these advantages, I managed to convince myself that since everything I served my kids was "clean label," I wasn't doing any harm. But of course, whether it's made from organic, whole-muscle meat or chopped up who-knows-what, a chicken nugget is a chicken nugget to a child's developing palate. These "kids' meals" were only making their acceptance of healthier food that much harder.

By the time I launched *The Lunch Tray*, our kids were eight and ten, and getting them to regularly eat fruits and vegetables was often still a struggle. So I selfishly exploited my new blogging platform to connect with some of the country's leading child feeding experts, hoping to cadge a little personalized advice as I interviewed them. From those discussions and the additional research I undertook for this book, I can now see with painful clarity every feeding pitfall I fell into when my kids were little. And in speaking with a lot of other frustrated parents over the years, I know I'm hardly alone in having made these mistakes.

Take Justin, the dad quoted above whose daughter will only eat the "Brown Food Diet." According to him, it didn't start out that way. "When she was born," he told me, "I had every intention of teaching her to eat well. I made all her purées from scratch and she ate just about anything I put in front of her." All of that changed, however, when she first started eating finger foods. (Does this sound familiar?) Because Justin was his family's designated cook, dinner time tended to be on the late side due to his work schedule and that created its own problems. "Tired of a whining and hungry toddler," he told me, "my wife would open the freezer where I kept lots of foods my daughter liked, and go, 'What do you want to eat?' and just feed her dinner. That got her used to eating on *her* schedule, not ours, and also to ordering up her favorite foods like it's a restaurant."

Fast forward to today, when Justin's daughter is six, and mealtimes are stressful for everyone. "We play the 'Please try a bite . . . no a *whole* bite, don't just stick it on your tongue' game, and the 'You can only have this if you eat three bites of that first' game, and every other tug-of-war-over-the-plate game that's ever been played by parents." Yet his daughter remains stubbornly resistant. "It pisses me off," Justin said candidly. "I was determined not to let that happen, but here we are."

Justin's feelings of anger and frustration are typical, says Dr. Lucy Cooke. She's a psychologist and child-feeding expert at University College London, but also the parent of now-grown, formerly picky children. "It's such an emotive thing, getting enough food into your child," she recalls. "I ran around in circles making special meals for them, not feeding them the same things I was eating, and resorting to all sorts of processed bits and bobs. You find yourself caving in and serving whatever will get eaten."

That's definitely been the case for Melissa,* a mom in Madison, Wisconsin, who struggles daily with feeding her two sons. Both are selective eaters who stubbornly stick to a limited range of familiar, bland foods like noodles, chicken nuggets, and yogurt. So Melissa, who's also the family's primary breadwinner, exhausts herself each night by playing short-order cook to satisfy everyone's demands. "We're in this scenario where I'm cooking three different meals," she confessed, "because I'm not eating buttered noodles every night."

Even being a registered dietician didn't prevent Katie, a mom of two living in a Houston suburb, from having a child who resists healthier food. "She's addicted to anything in a box," Katie lamented. "She could be starving all day and still turn her up her nose at an entire dinner, but I literally had to put a baby gate on the pantry because she'll eat her weight in Goldfish. She will never turn down a graham cracker, Goldfish, Cheez-Its—anything in a wrapper."

These parents are all fortunate enough to have regular access to fresh, whole foods, even if those foods are often spurned by their children. For millions of low-income families, feeding kids healthfully is even more challenging. On a calorie-for-dollar basis, highly processed food is usually the better bargain for cash-strapped parents, especially as compared to fresh produce. And while processed food and fast food are available almost everywhere, healthier food can be frustratingly hard to come by in less affluent neighborhoods: In more than half the ZIP codes in America in which the median annual income is under $25,000, there isn't a single supermarket nearby. When families have to travel farther to shop, they typically do so less often, which creates yet another disincentive to keep healthier (but often perishable) food at home. And many parents don't have access to a car, which has been identified as one of the most important factors in shaping a family's diet.

But even when parents do have access to healthy food, and even when they have every intention of raising healthy eaters, many still wind up feeling defeated. How exactly does that happen, and how can parents better instill in their kids a love of healthier food? I don't hold myself out as a credentialed expert in the field (and in this book's Appendix you'll

---

* Name changed at the interviewee's request.

find excellent books and resources from some of the best), but here's the low-down on everything I wish I'd known about feeding kids *before* I became a mom.

## Is It Pickiness—Or Just Being a Kid?

First, like many parents, I now realize I was too quick to assume that my son was a "picky eater" whose veggie-avoidance was a "problem" that had to be affirmatively "solved." After all, when a child is slow to reach other developmental milestones, like mastering potty-training or giving up thumb-sucking, we parents usually see those delays for what they are—temporary bumps in the road—instead of as ingrained personality traits that will forever define our children. But when it comes to eating, for some reason too many of us immediately slap the "picky eater" label on our child, which can fundamentally change what we feed them and how we interact with them at mealtimes.

I also had no idea that *all* children go through a least some period of "food neophobia" (a fear of trying new foods), a behavior that typically crops up in late infancy or toddlerhood. In other words, my son and Justin's daughter were right on schedule. Yet for uninformed parents (read: most of us), this sudden rejection of new foods can feel like it comes out of nowhere, especially since it often follows a period in which a baby happily eats anything and everything.

Food neophobia can leave parents frustrated and confused, but it's actually a beneficial holdover from our plant-foraging past. Children's small bodies are especially vulnerable to toxins, so it makes good sense for them to become extra-cautious about new foods once they can escape adults' watchful eyes. And here's a fun fact supporting this evolutionary theory: Other plant-eating animals, including gorillas, rats, and fish, also experience food neophobia around the time they emerge from infancy. (I find it oddly comforting to know that even gorilla moms have to deal with picky offspring.)

With respect to vegetables specifically, I also learned that all kids are hardwired at birth to have an aversion to bitter flavors, likely because bitterness is a clear signal in the wild that a plant might be poisonous. Many healthy vegetables also contain bitter flavor notes, so it makes sense that these foods can be among the hardest for many kids to accept. And some children are also "super-tasters," meaning they're even more sensitive to bitterness in foods. (When our son later took a super-taster test in science class, we weren't remotely surprised by the result.)

The majority of kids outgrow these innate behaviors, but some children are in fact genetically predisposed to be more selective when it comes to food. This is especially true if they're prone to anxiety and shyness. (Melissa, the mom from Madison, mentioned that one of her sons has generalized anxiety disorder.) The genetic link for selective eating has also been found to be strongest for more palate-challenging foods like fruits, vegetables, and proteins, while kids' preferences for snacks, starches, and dairy appear to be more influenced by their environment.

Meanwhile, just as adults are hardwired to seek out calorie-dense foods rich in salt, sugar, and fat, the same is true of kids. But as many frustrated parents have long suspected, there are real, biological reasons why children might be even more drawn than adults to highly processed foods.

Let's start with kids' love of sugar, which is evident even before they're born: If there's an influx of sweetness in the amniotic fluid, a fetus will immediately respond with increased swallowing. This trait primes babies to seek out their mother's naturally sweet breast milk, as well as sweet foods in the wild which tend to have the calorie-density needed for growth. But kids' love of sugar is so powerful, they'll eat foods that make Mother Nature's sweetest offerings pale in comparison. For example, most adults find cola—with its seven teaspoons of sugar per glass—sufficiently sweet, but kids will happily drink a glass containing *twelve* teaspoons. Consistent with its evolutionary purpose, kids' tolerance for super-sweetness tends to peak during periods of rapid growth, dropping off to the level preferred by adults once teens reach their full height.

Sugar also triggers powerful emotional responses in children. For example, when babies are given a bit of sugar solution, their faces immediately relax, sometimes into a full smile. When a sweet solution is given to agitated babies, their heart rates decrease and they quickly calm down, while in calm babies, the reverse is true: a bit of sugary solution perks them up by increasing their heart rate. Sugar also has a pain-relieving effect in children, so much so that offering a bit of sugar solution or candy is now considered a safe and effective way to reduce a child's discomfort during painful procedures like a blood draw or circumcision.

Babies also have a "salt tooth," although it takes them about two months before they can detect salt on their tongues. Just as with sugar, a baby's attraction to salt is correlated with periods of growth (likely because it draws them to needed minerals in foods) and it can be intensified—possibly for life—if he's exposed to too much salt too soon. According to one study, if high-sodium foods like crackers, bread, or cereal are given to a baby before six months of age, he'll be significantly more likely even at age four to prefer savory snacks over sweet, and he may even be that kid who licks the salt off pretzels or eats salt directly from the shaker.

Put all of these factors together—an innate attraction to extra-sweet and salty foods, a tendency to dislike vegetables' bitterness, and a guaranteed period in late infancy or toddlerhood when new foods will be spurned—and it's easy to see why so many parents leap to the conclusion that they have a "picky eater" on their hands. In fact, researchers from the University of Tennessee found in 2004 that fully 50 percent of parents identified their two-year-old as "picky."

## Making Matters Worse

Whether responding to perceived pickiness or to a child who really is a more selective eater, parents can then compound the problem by limiting the foods they offer or regularly falling back on kid food—both of which can solidify behaviors that might otherwise have been a passing phase.* Indeed, the University of Tennessee study found that many parents give up on offering a new food after just three to five exposures, even though kids may need up to fifteen before accepting it. More recently, a poll of two thousand British parents found that half were so frustrated by their children's resistance to fruits and vegetables, they'd simply given up on trying to get their kids to eat their daily recommended servings of these healthy foods.

---

* When I refer to "picky eating" in this book, I'm not speaking of the more extreme eating behaviors that fall under the rubric of "avoidant/restrictive food intake disorder" (ARFID). For parents who suspect their child may have ARFID, be sure to consult the "Picky Eating" section in this book's Appendix.

Picky eating can also be exacerbated by socioeconomics. In a two-year study of more than seventy families, a Harvard researcher found that lower-income parents often feel they can't afford to keep buying the healthy foods their kids are likely to reject, so they reluctantly fall back on the highly processed foods they love. As a result, lower-income kids may get fewer opportunities to even try challenging but healthy foods, while children in more affluent families are more likely to get the multiple exposures they need to overcome their initial reluctance.

Parents' income level can also affect their children's eating habits in less obvious ways. A recent study found that lower-income parents were just as concerned about their kids' health as more affluent parents, but they were far less likely to deny their children's request for unhealthy products. (Thirteen percent of low-income parents reported regularly saying "no," as compared to 96 percent of more affluent parents.) According to the researchers, more affluent parents derive a sense of self-worth by cultivating in their kids a taste for healthy food and by transmitting the "right" food values; for parents of lesser means, saying "yes" to unhealthy food offers a rare opportunity to indulge their kids, which in turn bolsters their sense of self-worth as a provider.

Whatever the reason, when parents fall back on offering highly processed foods, with all their carefully engineered deliciousness, children often become even less inclined to eat the healthy stuff. As sociologist and child-feeding expert Dr. Dina Rose explained to me, "Fresh fruits and vegetables don't seem like their processed cousins. Baked chicken doesn't seem like chicken nuggets." As a result, she says, parents need to factor in not just the relative healthfulness (or lack thereof) of processed foods, but also the fact that these salty, sugary, fatty flavors inevitably "push kids' taste preferences toward junk."

Yet if parents are at times too quick to stop offering healthier foods, it's also possible to veer too far in the other direction. More authoritarian parents, the ones who push their kids to eat unwanted foods, may wind up reinforcing the very behavior they're trying to curb. In one well-known study, a group of preschoolers was offered a small cup of soup and allowed to eat it or not, while a second group was repeatedly pressured by the experimenter to "finish your soup." The outcome was remarkable: kids in the pressured group were overwhelmingly negative in their comments about the soup—lots of "yucks" and "I'm not going to eat it"—as compared to the control group.

It's not just heavy-handed techniques like demanding a clean plate that can backfire. Even gentle pressure that seems benign to adults, like my ill-conceived sticker charts, offering a food reward ("No dessert until you eat your vegetables!"), or making children take a "no thank you" bite, can all increase a child's dislike of a given food. By this standard, every one of the dinner table "games" Justin and his wife engage in with their daughter would be considered counterproductive pressure. In fact, just telling a child how nutritious a food is, which many parents view as only instructive and encouraging, can lead a reluctant eater to view the food unfavorably or make her feel pressured.

Clearly, there are *a lot* of ways parents can muck up child feeding without meaning to. And our mistakes can start piling up even earlier than we might realize.

## Those First Tiny Tastes

Let's dial back the clock to when parents first introduce solid foods. Remember how babies look content and may even smile in response to sweet foods? Well, kids have automatic responses to other flavors as well, and sometimes those responses can mislead parents. As Cooke, the London psychologist, explained to me, "There are certain characteristic facial expressions in response to sweet, sour, and bitter flavors, which you can also see in primates—and even rat pups. So when you give a baby a strongly flavored vegetable, or sour things like lemons, they make these funny faces and parents get a bit put off," sometimes wrongly concluding the child dislikes the flavor. That's even more likely when a parent is herself a selective eater, which may predispose her to misinterpret that wrinkled nose or tiny scowl as outright rejection.

Then there's the question of how and when solids are first introduced. When my kids were babies, the prevailing advice was to wait until they were six months old and to start with iron-fortified white rice cereal, which was considered the "ideal" first food. Then you were supposed to introduce puréed fruits and vegetables, just one at a time and with a wait of several days between each, to ensure there were no allergic reactions.

But it turns out this super-cautious approach may not be the best way to prevent food allergies; more recent research indicates that for kids at high risk of developing a peanut allergy, an *earlier* introduction of peanuts is more effective. On top of that, this feeding advice could actually predispose a child to become a picky eater.

First, white rice cereal is one of the blandest foods on the planet, which means it does nothing to familiarize babies with more challenging flavors—and it might even instill in kids a lifelong preference for unhealthy, refined carbohydrates. That's the view of Stanford University pediatrician Alan Greene, who calls rice cereal "the taproot of childhood obesity" and started the "White Out" movement in 2011 to get doctors and parents to rethink its longstanding reputation the best first food. Rice cereal may also contain excessive amounts of naturally occurring arsenic, which is why the American Academy of Pediatrics now recommends that parents offer a wider variety of iron-fortified, whole-grain cereals, including oat, wheat, and barley.

Bland cereal aside, we also now know there's a "flavor window" during which babies are especially receptive to new tastes. And although that window doesn't close until around eighteen months, the optimal period for accepting new flavors is between four and six months, right when many babies are still consuming only breast milk or formula. It's also been found that babies' overall willingness to accept new flavors during this narrower window actually increases when they're exposed to a wider variety of new tastes, such as offering a different puréed vegetable each day. So by waiting until six months to introduce solid foods and then slowly introducing just one food at a time, as is still advised by many pediatricians, a parent may be squandering a lot of valuable "window time" that could have expanded his child's palate for life.*

Another early feeding pitfall is offering too many prepared baby and toddler foods that combine vegetables with sweet fruits. For example, among Beechnut's current line of toddler squeeze pouches, all but two of

---

* It goes without saying that a baby also needs to be developmentally ready to accept solid foods, meaning she: has roughly doubled her birth weight; can sit up with support; has good neck control; has a diminished tongue-thrust reflex (which automatically pushes food out of the mouth); and seems interested in solid food.

the vegetables are offered in fruit blends, like the rather odd combination of zucchini, spinach, and banana. Similarly, the only single-vegetable squeeze pouch offered by Plum Organics is one that's already sweet— sweet potato—and the rest are in blends like apple, spinach, and avocado. "That's a particular loathing of mine," Cooke says. "They'll never leave a vegetable alone, and they lead parents into thinking babies will only accept food if it's been sweetened in some way, which is complete non-sense." Few adults will ever eat broccoli and pear mixed together, she notes, yet "the manufacturer thinks, 'Well, the baby's not going to like broccoli so much if it's not sweet.' But obviously if you only ever serve them broccoli sweetened with pear, they'll struggle with broccoli on its own later on."

## What Mom Eats

Now dial the clock back further, to when a mom is still pregnant. It turns out that at around ten or eleven weeks, fetuses start to swallow amniotic fluid, which contains flavor molecules from their mother's diet. This means that the foods a pregnant mom eats regularly can actually shape her baby's later taste preferences, at least to some degree. In one study, when moms frequently drank carrot juice during their third trimester of pregnancy, their babies were more likely to later accept cereal prepared with carrot juice. The same effect has been found for flavors like vanilla, anise, garlic, and mint.

One way to look at this phenomenon is that it's nature's way of pre-paring a baby to accept whatever foods are normally eaten by the family or community she's about to join. But the darker side of this finding is that if a mother eats a poor diet during pregnancy, like one low in fruits and vegetables and heavy on the processed food, it could potentially cause her child to prefer a similarly unhealthy diet. While not yet replicated in humans, one study found that if a pregnant rat was fed an energy-dense, nutrient-poor and highly palatable diet (in other words, the rat equiva-lent of junk food), it actually altered the pleasure centers in her offspring's brains, causing them to overeat those foods in later life. So for low-in-come kids in particular, a mom's poor prenatal diet may be yet one more barrier to healthy eating.

Along these same lines, a mother's diet also shapes her baby's taste preferences through breastfeeding, since the flavor of her milk changes constantly based on what she eats. So in that same carrot juice study, when a separate group of moms drank the juice during the first two months of nursing (but not during pregnancy), their babies still were more likely to later accept the cereal made with carrot juice. By the same token, formula-fed babies are less likely to embrace new tastes because they've been exposed to just one flavor at every feeding. This is especially true if their formula is the more common cow milk-based variety, which has a bland flavor, as opposed to the strongly flavored, hydrolyzed-protein formula fed to babies with milk allergies.

There's another reason, too, why breastfed babies may be more open to new foods. Just as pressure at the dinner table can backfire, parents can see how much formula is left in a bottle and may unconsciously push formula-fed babies to drink more than needed to satisfy their hunger; breastfeeding, on the other hand, is child-led. These findings point to yet another way in which lower-income kids may lose out, since their mother's workplace is likely to be less supportive of breastfeeding than those of women in white collar jobs.

I take no joy in sharing information like this, because unless it's presented in a book on pregnancy or infant care, it usually comes too late for most parents and only leaves them feeling defeated. In my case, when I first learned about the "flavor window" from Bee Wilson's excellent book *First Bite: How We Learn to Eat*, I actually put my head in my hands and groaned. Who knows if it would have made any difference, but I can't help but picture my son, now a teenager, diving into salads with gusto if only I'd dabbed a bunch of puréed vegetables on his tiny tongue when he was four months old.

For the record, though, my son does now enjoy some vegetables, and what I've learned the hard way is that his continuing embrace of new foods has to happen on *his* timetable and at his initiation. Encountering dreaded mushrooms in an otherwise delicious ethnic dish led to that first tentative nibble, while enjoying deep-fried cauliflower at a restaurant opened the door to eating roasted cauliflower at home. I try not to insert myself in these developments, even to offer praise, instead just noting them out of the corner of my eye while silently cheering him on.

# Giving Kids a Chance to Learn

Putting kids in the driver's seat is at the heart of a child-feeding model that's almost universally recognized as the best way to raise confident, competent eaters. Called the "Division of Responsibility" (DOR), this approach gives parents sole responsibility for deciding what children will eat and when they'll eat it, while children are solely responsible for deciding whether to eat and how much. First proposed by renowned child-feeding expert and family therapist Ellyn Satter, the idea behind the DOR is that children have both the capacity and drive to model their parents' eating behavior, and they'll naturally do so—if allowed to learn at their own pace and without any adult pressure.

Granted, on parents' side of the DOR, there are some critical obligations: providing children with nutritious food in a structured eating environment—the "what" and "when" of eating—which means scheduled snacks and meals instead of unfettered grazing. It also means no jumping up to grab Cheerios or a yogurt tube when your child rejects the evening's entrée. As Satter puts it bluntly: "She is growing up to join you at your family table; you are not learning to eat off the high-chair tray."

Ideally, the DOR also requires that the child and at least one parent sit down to the same meal, because a key component is giving children a chance to observe their parents' eating behavior. This modeling does make a real difference: in one study, preschoolers were more likely to eat a colored porridge with an unfamiliar flavor if they were seated with a trusted adult who enthusiastically ate porridge of the same color. Similarly, many species of young animals have been observed taking cues from their elders before trying new foods.

And yet for a lot of parents, so many necessary components of the DOR can feel hopelessly out of reach. Or, as Justin put it, "It's easy enough to say, 'You all need to sit down at the table for a meal and she has to eat what's served or starve,' but it just doesn't always work out that easy."

For one thing, as is the case in Justin's family, 70 percent of moms now work outside the home, and with both parents working it can be hard to find the time for meal planning, grocery shopping, and cooking. Indeed, according to one study of millennial mothers, 80 percent said they usually don't know what they're serving for dinner until late in the afternoon. Not coincidentally, the number of restaurants and fast food chains has grown exponentially since the 1970s, when women first began to join the workforce in greater numbers. And for lower-income parents working more than one job, the prospect of home cooking can be not only daunting but seemingly impossible.

Kids' schedules, too, are more packed than ever. A recent Pew report found that three-fourths of school-aged kids had participated in sports in the prior year, while over half had participated in other extracurricular activities, all of which can get in the way of dining together at home. This may explain why, according to that same millennial moms study, one out of five meals eaten by kids are consumed in a car.

Cooking is also generally on the decline, with many of today's parents having been raised by parents who didn't regularly prepare meals from scratch, depriving them of the opportunity to learn by observation. And while a lot of people used to learn basic cooking skills in home economics classes at school, that instruction is virtually nonexistent today. So despite America's current love affair with cooking shows, fewer parents than ever are able to offer home-cooked meals to their families.

Of course, a meal doesn't have to be prepared from scratch to count as family dinner; gathering around the table to eat restaurant take-out or a bowl of pasta and jarred sauce still offers children a chance to observe adult eating. The problem, however, is that a heavy reliance on highly processed food can actually *interfere* with family members all sitting down together—even when they're able to do so. That was the surprising finding of the UCLA Sloan Center on Everyday Lives of Families (CELF), which intensively studied the daily lives of thirty-two middle class, dual-income families in the early 2000s.

The CELF researchers were initially surprised to learn that 73 percent of the dinners eaten by these families were reportedly "home-cooked." But when they dug deeper, they learned that only 22 percent of these meals were actually prepared from fresh ingredients, while the rest were composed of highly processed foods like frozen Trader Joe's orange chicken, frozen French fries, ramen soups, and Rice-A-Roni. Putting aside any nutritional concerns about those foods, when the researchers matched the contents of a given meal to the manner in which it was eaten, they found a strong correlation between a reliance on processed foods and disjointed dining experiences in which family members ate in different rooms or at different times, even when they were all at home at the same time. In contrast, when a meal was prepared mainly with fresh ingredients, the family was far more likely to sit down and eat together.

The same effect was seen with snacking. Today's kids eat between meals far more frequently than previous generations, with most now eating snacks three times a day, and some doing so as many as six times per day. That habit alone can keep kids from coming to the table hungry, a prerequisite to learning good eating habits. But the CELF researchers also noted that today's families typically stock their pantries with a lot of highly processed items, including individual-sized snack packs and easy-to-prepare, single portion meals—all of which, in the researchers' words, make it even easier for kids to "eat at will and apart."

And even when snacks are healthy, they can still exacerbate picky eating if kids are allowed to graze on them all day. Take those toddler squeeze pouches I mentioned earlier. It's hard to remember a time when kids weren't contentedly sucking on puréed food in their strollers and car seats, but the squeeze pouch is the relatively recent invention of Neil Grimmer, the CEO of Plum Organics. He created a prototype to get his own children to eat fruits and vegetables, but his idea turned out to be revolutionary: Plum Organics's pouch revenues reportedly skyrocketed from $4,800 in 2008 to $53 million within just four years. Grimmer's competitors quickly followed suit, and today almost one-third of all baby food is eaten from a pouch, even though it retails for nearly twice as much as puréed food in a jar.

Not having to worry about spoons or spills is a boon for on-the-go families, and pouches also give older babies and toddlers more independence in feeding themselves. But putting aside other concerns about puréed fruit blends (particularly their lower fiber-to-sugar ratio and the fact that they don't teach kids how to chew), this very independence and lack of structure around eating can quickly undermine the DOR. As Carol Danaher, a public health nutritionist and board president of the Ellyn Satter Institute, puts it, "Routinely letting the child eat from pouches on the run, whenever she wants, is an abrogation of one of the most basic of parenting roles—providing the child with a predictable routine for meals and snacks. It also doesn't help the child learn to eat the family foods."

## Holding the Line

This leads us to yet another factor that gets in the way of the DOR: the arguably too-permissive parenting style of many of today's parents. In order to impose any kind of structure on a child's eating, a parent has to be willing to withstand the inevitable blowback when, for example, the child wants a huge snack right before dinner, or begs for alternate, kid-friendly food when she doesn't like what's being served. Yet many parents are very uncomfortable imposing that kind of discipline. In recalling her experience teaching a DOR-based feeding class to parents of varying income levels and from different cultures, Danaher found that "this was a really common behavior. Parents just couldn't stand up to their child's crying or begging for certain snacks or foods so they would just give in, thus undermining the structure and routines that they wished to provide."

Cooke understands why parents may balk. "To let your child go to bed hungry, or to go to school hungry, that's a really hard one. I'm very sympathetic to parents who cave in," she says. "I'm all about empowering them to be a bit braver." And some parents may simply prefer to "hold their fire" for more serious infractions instead of imposing discipline around eating. As Cooke recalled from her own days as a parent of picky children, "I was quite an authoritative parent about many things, like manners, but I know I wasn't particularly authoritative about food. Parenting tends to be quite domain-specific, and parents can be quite permissive in certain areas and not in others."

For better or worse, there's clearly been a sea-change in parents' deference to children at mealtimes. Consider this guidance on handling picky eating from a 1825 parenting treatise—advice that's about as scarily authoritarian as it gets: "[The child] is not to think for itself. Neither its palate nor its caprice is to be consulted—the parent must set before it for its meals, such articles of food as are judged best for it, and it is to be made to understand, that it must eat them, or nothing." Whatever you think of that approach (not to mention the use of "it" to refer to a child!), contrast it with this all-too-familiar parent-child exchange about dinner, documented by the CELF researchers. Susan is the mom and Courtney is her eight-year-old daughter:

> SUSAN: Hey lounge lizard.
> COURTNEY: (Hello.)
> SUSAN: You want, um—want something to eat?
> COURTNEY: No. I don't like [name of restaurant.]
> SUSAN: I didn't get [name of restaurant], and what are you eating now? Goldfish again?
> COURTNEY: [nods]
> SUSAN: So what do you want? Salad and a quesadilla?
> COURTNEY: [shakes her head]
> SUSAN: Come on. [pause] What do you want to eat? I'll make you something and then we're turning off the TV, Courtney.
> SUSAN: What do you want to eat?
> COURTNEY: I don't want anything.
> SUSAN: You don't want, um [pause] a salad or an apple or [pause] what.
> COURTNEY: [shakes her head]

Not only do today's parents cede an unprecedented amount of control to their children over the foods served at mealtime, they also give kids far more say in the grocery store. One recent study actually found that kids' taste preferences influenced 95 *percent* of parents' food and beverage purchase decisions. Letting kids choose between parent-approved foods is fine ("Would you rather have green beans with dinner, or corn on the cob?") but when kids start making baseline decisions about the entire family's diet, it's a clear violation of the DOR. As Satter reminds parents who waver on this issue: "You know more about the food in the world than she does."

But if you only have a few hours a day with your child before she has to dive into homework and go to bed, who wants to spend that precious time in conflict over eating? As Cooke observes, "Working mums may be feeling guilty about not being with their kids so much. So when they are at home, they indulge them a bit more." Melissa, the working mom in Madison with two picky sons, is a perfect example. In explaining to me the many nutritional compromises she's made over the years, she repeatedly referred to an overarching desire to keep the peace with her children. "That's why you settle on the processed food," she said. "It means not fighting about it all the time, and setting up some harmful parenting relationship. It's a soft place to land."

Even when parents knowingly make these trade-offs, however, they don't always feel good about them. "There's a lot of pressure to get food in them that's not fast food or whatever," Melissa says with regret. "If I were a stay-at-home mom, I'd like to think I'd be doing a better job." But I was quick to reassure Melissa that I *was* a stay-at-home mom and still experienced a lot of the same guilt and worry. I saw nourishing my children as one of my most important responsibilities, so when they spurned healthier food, I felt like a failure. I was concerned about their health, too; with each rejected carrot stick and apple slice, I would mentally rack up in my head all the nutrients they weren't getting on a regular basis. I also felt intense frustration when my kids sometimes refused to take a single bite of a dish before rejecting it, especially since I'd put a fair amount of time and effort into shopping for and preparing the meal.

That heady swirl of negative emotions—anger, fear, guilt, and worry—is what marketers cynically refer to as a "pain point." And whenever an industry sniffs one of these out, it also smells the enticing aroma of potential profits. It's a fear of disease, after all, that drives the sale of hand sanitizers, and the fear of being socially ostracized that sells deodorant and mouthwash. But the exploitation of this particular pain point—one that's keenly felt by so many parents across the country—produces a perverse result: the processed food industry winds up promoting its products as the "solution" to children's unhealthy eating habits, even though so many of these products are actually a significant driver of the problem.

The industry pulls off this sleight of hand with a two-pronged approach: breaking down parents' ability to act as good dietary gatekeepers, while simultaneously stoking kids' desire for the least healthy foods. As we're about to see, it's a powerfully effective divide-and-conquer strategy that lines corporate coffers—even as children pay the real price.

# 3

# THE CLAIM GAME

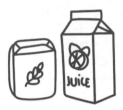

*I think we're an easy target for the industry. We're just kind of ripe for the picking.*

~ MOM OF TWO, MADISON, WISCONSIN

Every parent has been there: that moment when you grudgingly toss into your grocery cart a product you suspect isn't so great for your kids, but:

(a) You've learned from bitter experience it's the only brand they'll eat,

(b) It says on the box that it "contains calcium and vitamin C," and you're just going to go with that,

(c) You made the mistake of grocery shopping with your children at 5 p.m., you've already said "no" to ten other products, and you can't take another second of nagging,

(d) All of the above, and please stop asking questions—one of the
kids is having a major meltdown in aisle 9.

Food and beverage companies know that parents—well, mostly
mothers, according to statistics—are the ultimate decision makers in the
supermarket, and they'll do pretty much anything to win them over. Or
as Dan Parker, a former British ad executive, explained to me: "There's an
expression in the industry, which is, 'What's in it for Mum?' On every
piece of material you create, whether it's packaging or an ad or whatever,
you always ask the question, 'What's here for Mum?'"

Parker knows what he's talking about. For more than two decades, he
helped market some of the biggest names in the industry, including
Coca-Cola, McDonald's, Cadbury, and PepsiCo. Or, in his words, "Lots
of snacks, lots of fizzy drinks, lots of junk food." Yet Parker had no qualms
about using his talents to convince the rest of us to buy these unhealthy
products. "I was young, arrogant, and ignorant," he says. "And if someone's
a brand manager on Coca-Cola and they're twenty-seven, earning a hundred thousand dollars a year, and they get invited to every cool party in
town, these people end up pretty blinkered, don't they? We spent our
lives in expensive bars and clubs, drinking champagne and eating nice
food, and we didn't really see the real world."

But in 2014, the real world harshly intruded on Parker: he learned
he'd developed type 2 diabetes, the same disease that had killed his father.
"My dad was quite obese," Parker recalls, "and he had twenty years of
misery before he died. My wife never knew a version of my dad who
wasn't miserable, and I have to say, even I have to think really hard to remember one."

Faced with this frightening diagnosis and now also a father himself,
Parker resolved to turn his life around. He shuttered his marketing
agency and started a nonprofit, Living Loud, dedicated to improving the
diets and health of UK citizens. He's since testified before the House of
Commons about childhood obesity, consulted with celebrity chef Jamie
Oliver on a nationwide campaign to reduce sugar consumption, and
become a vocal critic of his former Big Food clients.

When I first learned about Parker on social media, his story resonated. That's because I, too, used to work in the belly of the beast, as a

senior in-house marketing attorney for Unilever. This multinational food and consumer products conglomerate isn't a household name here in America, but it owns hundreds of iconic brands like Popsicle, Ben & Jerry's, Lipton, and Ragú. It was my job to sign off on the package copy and ad campaigns developed by people like Parker, and my four years at the company showed me exactly how marketers try to influence consumers—and how they try to push the envelope.

"As a creative director, I spent my life dealing with people like yourself," Parker told me. "I would come up with an idea, and you'd say, 'That's a little over the line,' and eventually I would push up to the absolute edge of what you would allow me to do." As Parker sees it, it's inevitable that advertisers will test the law's outer limits. "It's an incredibly competitive marketplace," he says. "You've got these hugely powerful corporations, and then you've got literally thousands of companies that would like to supply them with [marketing] work. And the way to compete in the world of advertising is you have to push to the absolute edges of acceptability."

## How the Game Is Played

Seeing through marketing ploys is the first step in arming yourself against them. So let's take a closer look at how marketers capitalize on parents' frustrations and concerns about their children's eating, from relatively harmless persuasion to the tactics that skirt the "absolute edge."

### We Can Get (Unhealthy) Food into Your Kid!

Food companies know just how exhausting it can be to get a meal on the table—and how maddening it is when a child spurns it. So they're all too happy to exploit that frustration by promising their products will never, ever be rejected.

Tyson Foods, king of the kid-friendly chicken nugget, is a particular fan of this approach. In one of its ads, a mom goes to ridiculous extremes to please her children at dinner, like hiring a circus act and making food sculptures, until she wins them over with the company's fried chicken strips. Another Tyson ad showed picky kids poking at their meals, classifying each child as "the rejecter," "the inspector," and the "no thank you."

(Good thing its dinosaur-shaped nuggets are the "fun way to a clean plate!") Tyson also once had children address the camera with a list of all the foods they hate, while an announcer reassured parents that Tyson nuggets are "the one thing kids love 100 percent of the time!"

But Tyson is hardly the only company using this approach. Kellogg's once ran a commercial showing a boy turning down every breakfast his mom offers, until she discovers that Eggo waffles "win over the pickiest eaters!" Ore-Ida even recently encouraged parents, in a way that was tongue-in-cheek but also kind of *not*, to reward kids with the company's French fries for choking down healthy foods like carrots and Brussels sprouts.

When it comes to obviously unhealthy products like fried chicken and French fries, it's hard to argue anyone's being duped. Instead, these pitches work because they're a siren song for stressed-out parents: "Just give your kids the less-healthy food they *really* want. We won't tell."

### Our (Unhealthy) Food Will Buy Some Peace and Quiet!

Getting kids to sit down and behave at dinner is a challenge for some parents, so why not let junk food do the "disciplining" for you?

That's another classic industry pitch, like the Kid Cuisine frozen meal promising that "colossal hunks of Popcorn Chicken and super colorful sprinkles to mix in [the] pudding" will "restore peace and order to your dinner table." A 2019 Kraft Heinz ad showed an annoyed dad silencing his noisy daughters by offering mac and cheese: "You love how peaceful it is while they eat every bite. Finally, the marching band has stopped for just a few beautiful moments." A sugary toddler nutrition drink promises to "restore order at the dinner table" and end "mealtime chaos," while a harried mom in a KFC ad told viewers that without the chain's fried chicken tenders, "it's almost impossible to get them to sit down at dinner. . . . I cannot get these kids to eat anything, and right now? . . . Silence . . . I mean, he's sitting still. This is kind of miraculous."

Now if only that fried chicken could get your kid to clean his room. . . .

### Abandon Hope: Your Kid Will Never Accept Healthier Food!

If parents know picky eating is just a passing phase, they can grit their teeth and ride it out. But if it's an immutable trait shared by all children, what's the point in even trying to serve healthy food, right?

Kraft Heinz aggressively relied on this insidious messaging in 2019, showing kids running from broccoli and gagging at the sight of salmon until their parents swapped out their healthier dinners for mac and cheese. A Chef Boyardee campaign in 2010 sarcastically mocked pictures of children enjoying healthy food, with copy like "Behold the mythical veggie-loving kid. He doesn't exist" and "Oh, look. A Mother's Daydream. It'll never be a reality." And a toddler nutrition drink promises to provide the nutrients in foods "kids won't eat"—including "fish, spinach [and] broccoli"[4]—while a sugary snack bar states unequivocally that "kids don't like healthier food" because eating healthy isn't "fun."

### Our Packaging Is Tasteful, So Our Product Must Be Healthy!

Have you ever bought a product at Whole Foods just because its packaging gave off a wholesome, New Age vibe—even when it's the kind of food you'd never buy in a supermarket?

Cheez-Its cheese crackers, for example, positively scream "Big Food" with their bright red box, while their competitor, Back to Nature cheese crackers, are subtly "healthwashed" via their brand name and a tastefully minimalist, earth-toned aesthetic. Yet the ingredients and nutritional profiles of both products are virtually identical: mostly empty calories.

If you tend to fall for this kind of thing, take comfort in knowing you're not alone. A recent focus group study found that parents really do assume that a product sporting bright colors and cartoon characters is less healthy, and the opposite for foods packaged in earth tones. If you're committed to buying organic or avoiding certain chemicals, choosing the Whole Foods–type version may make sense. But products like frosted toaster pastries and white-flour mac and cheese typically don't deserve the nutritional free pass many parents give them when they're 100 percent natural.

### Our Product Is (Sort of) Healthy!

When parents see the words "made with real fruit" on a product for kids, they may want to run in the other direction. That's because the term "real fruit" can legally include concentrated fruit purée, which is actually just a form of added sugar. So instead of providing health benefits, that "fruit" can actually make a product *less* healthy for your kids. (Also worth considering: if a "fruit" product is so highly processed that someone actually needs to *tell* you it's made with real fruit...well, I'm looking at you, Wildlicious Frosted Wild Berry Pop-Tarts.)

This "fruitwashing" claim is just one way manufacturers make their products seem healthier than they actually are. In fact, pretty much any "made with" claim should be regarded by parents as a nutritional red flag until proven otherwise, whether it's "made with whole grain"—which can mean just a bit of whole grain in an otherwise refined product—or "made with [fill in current 'superfood']," which can mean that little more than a fairy dusting of goji berries (or oat bran, or green tea extract, or whatever) is actually in the product. Another industry favorite: "yogurt-covered" or "Greek yogurt-covered," which sounds like the coated food has been given a nutritional boost, when instead it's usually been dunked in a mixture of sugar, palm oil, and a mere dash of dried yogurt powder.

Manufacturers can also create this oh-so-desirable "health halo" by claiming on the label that a product:

+ contains more of some nutrients ("calcium-rich"),
+ contains less of others ("25 percent less sodium"),
+ doesn't contain something we think we should avoid ("gluten free"),
+ offers quasi-drug-like benefits ("with probiotics to support gut health"), or
+ is "healthy," if it meets certain (outdated) nutritional criteria set by the Food and Drug Administration.

These kinds of claims are so effective that marketers can't seem to get enough of them. A recent study of baby and toddler foods, for example, found that 96 percent of the packages studied contained some type of nutrition messages, averaging almost six messages each. And the number of nutrition messages was actually higher on *less* healthy baby and toddler snack foods, proving writer Michael Pollan's adage that "If you're concerned about your health, you should probably avoid products that make health claims." A Nielsen study broke it down even further and found that parents are particularly swayed by "made with fruits and vegetables"– type claims on snack foods (though claims like "high in fiber" or "natural flavors" weren't far behind), and that parents willingly pay more for products that seem healthier.

Nutrition claims like these are legal if a company has proper substantiation, and some products making them actually are as healthy as they appear. But because of the way the federal rules are structured, other products are a lot closer to Welch's blueberry Fruit'n Yogurt snacks. Their packaging is dominated by huge picture of fresh blueberries—"real fruit"—being dunked in a sea of "creamy yogurt," along with claims that they: contain calcium and vitamins A, C, and D; are "gluten free" and "low fat"; and come in "80 calorie" pouches. Healthy and wholesome, right?

Now take a look at their actual ingredients, the first three of which are a form of added sugar:

> Fruit Center: Fruit Purée (White Grape, Pear, and Blueberry), Sugar, Corn Syrup, Modified Corn Starch, Pectin, Tri-Calcium Phosphate, Citric Acid, Sodium Citrate, Natural and Artificial Blueberry Flavor, Red 40 Lake, Blue 1 Lake, Yogurt Coating: Sugar, Palm Kernel Oil, Whey Powder, Nonfat Milk Powder, Yogurt Powder (Cultured Whey and Nonfat Milk), Vitamin A Palmitate, Ascorbic Acid (Vitamin C), Vitamin D3, Titanium Dioxide, Soy Lecithin, Vanilla, Coconut Oil, Carnauba Wax and Confectioner's Glaze (Lac-Resin).

In other words: the nutritional equivalent of vitamin-fortified gummy candy.

And here's the real kicker: At least one study indicates that products marketed for children are actually more likely than other products to have misleading front label claims—making parents' detective work in the grocery store that much harder.

### We Can Sneak (a Micron of) Veggies into Your Kid!

Remember that "veggie-sneaking" craze a few years ago, when popular cookbooks told parents how to slip black beans into their children's brownies and beets into their red velvet cupcakes? The food industry loves this "stealth health" gimmick, too—but more for the marketing claims it generates than for any nutritional boost it might offer kids.

My favorite example of the stealth health strategy is the Girl Scouts' Mango Creme sandwich cookie, which debuted in 2013 and promised to provide kids with "all the nutrient benefits of eating cranberries, pomegranates, oranges, grapes, and strawberries!" This eyebrow-raising claim was based on a smidge of dehydrated fruit powder in the cream filling—powder which, ironically, didn't contain mango. But could that powder magically transform white flour cookies, with 8 grams of fat and 11 grams of sugar per serving, into something healthy? The marketing ploy was widely criticized—one public health group even wrote a protest letter to the Girl Scouts of America, while Gawker's headline read: "The New Girl Scout Cookie Tastes Like BULLSHIT"—and Mango Cremes were quietly dropped from the Girl Scout cookie lineup the following year.

The Girl Scouts may have taken it a step too far, but the stealth health strategy is still catnip to marketers. That's because it satisfies two consumer needs: it makes parents feel better about buying the less-healthy but delicious processed foods their kids love, *and* they can feel somewhat better when actual fruits and vegetables later go untouched at the table.

The snack food Veggie Booty was a pioneer among these kinds of "healthified" products. Back in the late 1990s and early 2000s, the packaging for these vegetable-coated puffs promised the product was "Good for You," with "a phytonutrient blend" that provided "the vitamins and minerals needed for maximum nutrition." A lot of gullible parents (myself included) fell for those claims, believing the snack was—if not quite the same as giving your kid a salad—at least a reasonably healthy choice. Meanwhile, toddlers couldn't get enough of its melt-in-your-mouth texture, so much so that Veggie Booty became widely known among parents as "baby crack." In New York City, where I lived at the time, you could hardly pass a stroller without seeing little fingers and faces smeared with green dust.

After changing ownership and garnering negative press for making false statements about its fat content, Veggie Booty has toned down its marketing, including dropping that misleading "Good for You" claim.*

---

* The company's original owner had the temerity to tell a reporter that "Good For You" on another of its "healthified" products—Veggie Tings— was just a pat on the back for the consumer. As in: "You bought this bag—well, good for you!"

Still, fruit- or veggie-infused "puffs," "straws," and "melts" remain a huge product category for older babies and toddlers—and many of them are equally suspect.

Gerber, for example, sells a product for toddlers called Organic Farm Greens Veggie Crisps in which the only "farm greens"—dried spinach and kale—appear dead last in the ingredient list, likely explaining why none of the vitamins and minerals found in spinach and kale appear on their Nutrition Facts label. Similarly, Plum Organics's Super Puffs with Blueberry and Purple Sweet Potato don't include any vitamin C—notable, given that both blueberries and sweet potatoes are a good source of that nutrient. Yet few parents have the time to carefully compare the ingredient listing to the Nutrition Facts to figure any of this out, especially when shopping with a restless toddler in tow.

Snacks for older kids use the same strategy, like those ubiquitous "veggie straws" sold by a number of manufacturers, including Whole Foods, that look like pale yellow, green, and orange French fries. Bags for these snacks are almost always plastered with pictures of spinach, carrots, or tomatoes, yet they're basically veggie-colored potato starch. You may think few parents are fooled by this gimmick, but a quick Google search of "Are veggie straws healthy?" shows how deep the confusion runs. As a registered dietitian writing in the Washington Post recently reported, "I've met many parents who think that 'veggie sticks'... are the miracle they've been waiting for, because they can finally get their kids to eat vegetables."

Other stealth health products actually do offer more than a mere hint of fruit and vegetables, but often it's still not much. That Chef Boyardee campaign promising to sneak a "full serving of vegetables" into unsuspecting kids apparently based that claim on the canned pasta's tomato sauce. (The other vegetables it contained, carrots and onions, were used in such small amounts, they appeared after salt in the ingredient listing.) The popular Kidfresh line of frozen meals makes hidden vegetables its entire selling point, sneaking pureed cauliflower in the breading of its fried chicken nuggets and pureed carrots into its quesadilla. The brand OH YES! goes even further, somehow managing to cram twelve different fruits and vegetables into its frozen pizzas.

But let's get real. "Sneaky" foods like these may improve children's diets, but only in the narrowest possible way. Sure, kids may unwittingly gulp down a spoonful (maybe two, max?) of veggies, but if the veggie-delivery vehicle is cheese pizza or a bowl of mac and cheese—and if they don't even know the veggies are in there—why not just serve regular pizza and hand your child a vitamin pill?

### Our Sugary Drink Is Pediatrician-Recommended (Except Not Really)!

Stealth health products are appealing because they seem like an easy—sometimes suspiciously easy—nutritional insurance policy for kids. But if some parents can see through the most outrageous claims, like a snack puff masquerading as kale, it's harder to resist products offering that same nutritional insurance *and* which appear to be backed by science. It's just these kinds of quasi-medical claims that drive sales of "toddler milks" and children's "nutrition shakes," two related product categories that unfairly exploit parents' concerns to the fullest.

### Toddler Milks

If you've never heard of toddler milks (also called "toddler drinks," "growing-up milks," and "toddler formulas"), just know this: they have very little to do with toddlers' dietary needs and everything to do with the financial needs of the infant formula industry.

Thanks to increased rates of breastfeeding, infant formula manufacturers have taken a big hit in recent years. So now they're focusing on "life-stage targeting," which means promoting toddler products even more aggressively than those for babies: In 2015, the industry spent $9 million to market infant formulas and $16 million on toddler milks. And it's been money well spent. As of 2014, toddler beverages were a $15 billion business worldwide and the biggest and fastest-growing product sold by formula manufacturers. In fact, a recent study from the University of Connecticut's Rudd Center for Food Policy & Obesity suggests that more than 40 percent of American parents offer toddler drinks to their kids—in some cases, every day.

So what's the problem with toddler drinks? Because they're sold under trusted, pediatrician-approved brands like Gerber, Similac, and Enfagrow, usually with the same package design as their infant formulas, many parents mistakenly believe the drinks are just the next required step in formula feeding. Yet experts say these sugar-sweetened, vitamin-fortified blends of vegetable oil and powdered milk actually have no place in a child's healthy diet. Children under age one are only supposed to drink breast milk or formula, according to the American Academy of Pediatrics, yet some toddler beverages claim to be appropriate for babies as young as nine months. Meanwhile, toddlers over twelve months are supposed to be drinking whole, plain cow's milk, which has less sodium and more protein than typical toddler drinks. And based on American Heart Association guidelines, kids under two aren't supposed to consume any of the added sugars these drinks all contain.

Despite this clear expert consensus against the use of toddler beverages, the industry remains undeterred and unrepentant. Instead, because toddler drinks are far less regulated than formula, companies continue to make all kinds of questionable claims for them:

+ superlatives like "Number 1 brand recommended by pediatricians"— even though *no* major pediatric group recommends these products,
+ carefully worded, borderline-medical claims that prey on parents' fears, like "nourish[es] the development that helps your toddler reach milestones," or "now with Triple Health Guard," or
+ ominous-sounding warnings like "[t]he transition...to cow's milk can lead to a drop in brain-nourishing DHA consumption. That's why it's important to help promote your little one's brain development with...."

On top of all that, many toddler milks are also promoted to parents as a necessary countermeasure against children's picky eating, because they help "fill any nutritional gaps" or balance an "uneven" diet. Yet the irony is, experts say these products are likely to make a child's picky eating even worse.

According to pediatrician and registered dietitian Natalie Digate Muth, a sweet, filling toddler drink not only fails to provide any nutritional benefits over a multivitamin, it's usually offered "at the precise time that introduction of 'real food' is essential to avoid picky eating later." As a result, Muth says, these products are "a perfect example of short-term 'gain'—vitamins and minerals—for a long-term loss," and their use means "kids will stay picky for that much longer and miss out on the many benefits of eating a wide variety of healthful foods of various tastes and textures." She also notes that children may reject food because they're simply not hungry, so offering them a sweet drink may only teach them to ignore their own feelings of hunger and fullness.

This marketing ploy may be bad for kids, but it's a brilliant strategy for formula companies. All toddlers experience some fear of trying new foods, if not more generalized pickiness on top of that, and these eating behaviors tend to cause a lot of anxiety for parents. So, in essence, every parent becomes a potential target for this fear-mongering pitch.

*Nutrition Shakes*

Unlike toddler drinks, "nutrition shakes" for older children have been around for decades, and these high-calorie, nutrient-fortified drinks can be beneficial for underweight kids with eating disorders or other serious medical issues. But in 2010, the formula manufacturer Abbott Laboratories spotted a new marketing opportunity. It decided to expand its PediaSure brand of nutrition shakes to include SideKicks, a lower-calorie shake for older children that's meant "to help balance out a picky eater's uneven diet"—even if those kids are, in Abbott's words, "growing fine."

As a sugary, satiating beverage, SideKicks poses all the same problems as toddler milk when promoted as a "solution" for picky eating. Yet soon after the launch, Abbott created a "PediaSure Mom Brigade"— "mom dietitians" enlisted to convince other mothers their kids needed the product—while stressing the "significant emotional toll on moms" caused by picky eating. The company even ran a television spot that strongly implied kids who drink SideKicks are more active and energetic than kids who don't, and that they perform better in sports—a commercial Abbott was forced to pull after New York's Attorney General called it "false," "misleading," "exploitative" and "illegal." Indeed, the creative director behind this commercial showed unusual candor in describing on his own website the company's thinking behind it: "How do you convince moms to buy a sort-of-expensive nutritional drink for their kids? Good old-fashioned guilt."

That's all quite troubling, but it's nothing compared to how Abbott markets PediaSure outside the United States, particularly in Asia.

Sociologist Veronica Sau-Wa Mak, a lecturer at the Chinese University of Hong Kong, has intensively studied Abbott's years-long campaign in Hong Kong to first create and then stoke concern among Chinese parents about picky eating. A key strategy, she says, has been funding academic studies that "medicalize" children's picky eating behavior, studies which in turn influence pediatricians.

The effort has reportedly paid off. According to Mak, a 2003 survey found that only 28 percent of moms in Hong Kong were particularly worried about their children's health; most were primarily concerned with their children's academic performance. Less than ten years later, almost half of all parents of young children in Hong Kong said they felt worried about their children's picky eating habits, according to Mak, and the topic of picky eating became more widely discussed in local media.

My own review of Hong Kong advertising industry publications supports Mak's observations. In 2013, Abbott hired the Leo Burnett ad agency to promote PediaSure, and the agency came up with the slogan "Are You Sure?"—a needling question clearly meant to stoke moms' anxieties. In one article, Leo Burnett's group brand director said the slogan was part of its larger plan to market the product as "a holistic solution for kids' eating disorder syndrome." (Yikes—now picky eating is a "disorder" *and* a "syndrome"?) He also chastised the moms of Hong Kong for having "underestimated the impact of [picky eating] symptoms" and "see[ing] it as a different eating habit instead." Another advertising industry article noted that "[d]oting mothers in Hong Kong may not realize the danger of indulging their precious baby's picky-eating habits," and said the PediaSure campaign was meant to "confront mothers who may be unaware or in denial of such habits."

Burnett's spokesperson further observed, "Actually some moms are aware of this, but won't treat this as a 'problem.'" Imagine that.

## Generating Nutritional Noise

Few of the marketing pitches we've just discussed would be effective if parents weren't already conditioned to think about food in terms of its constituent ingredients instead of as a whole. Two hundred years ago, a cookie was a cookie; today, we're all more willing to let a manufacturer convince us it contains the same "nutrient benefits" as fruit.

This profound shift in thinking about food traces back to the nineteenth and early twentieth centuries, when the nutrients that make up food were first discovered. Since then, we've all become amateur food scientists, able to mentally break down our food into whatever components interest or concern us, whether it's fat, fiber, vitamins, or protein. This so-called "nutritionism" mindset is then reinforced by the latest studies linking diet to health and disease, which today are reported with such regularity that sometimes it feels like you need to hire an expert just to figure out what to feed your family. And when some of these widely publicized scientific findings are later reversed—I forget: do eggs cause heart attacks or are they healthy now?—we feel even less secure about our food choices.

It's no wonder, then, that we're all casting about for answers, whether it's shunning fat or cutting carbs. And even experts don't always agree. A 2016 survey found that ordinary Americans and registered dietitians easily concurred that apples and kale are healthy while soda and cookies aren't, but between those two extremes, things got a little hazy. The public overestimated the healthfulness of certain foods like orange juice, granola, and coconut oil (at least in the opinion of the dietitians), while the dietitians lauded foods about which ordinary people were uncertain, including quinoa, shrimp, and hummus. But the most telling finding was that neither the public *nor* the dietitians could agree over whether we ought to eat a lot of quite common foods—things like popcorn, butter, cheddar cheese, and pork chops.

No one is happier about this state of affairs than the processed food and beverage industries. As long as we remain unsure of the big picture and myopically focused on nutrients, companies only have to tweak their ingredients to profit off the latest dietary advice: if the market demands it, "low-fat" can become "paleo-friendly" overnight.

But these industries don't just take advantage of our food confusion— they also quite actively stoke it. So even as a dad is trying to figure out if that canister of toddler "veggie puffs" is as healthy as its packaging implies, corporations are spending millions each year to generally muddy the waters in the field of nutrition science—adding yet another layer of complexity and confusion in his decision-making. Here's how they create all that "nutritional noise":

*Studies (That We Paid For) Say Our Product's Healthy!*
*"Does candy keep kids from getting fat?"* That grabby headline appeared on one of several news stories back in 2011, reporting on a study finding that kids who eat candy have healthier body weights. For parents of candy-loving kids—that is to say, every parent, everywhere—this finding sounded almost too good to be true. And of course, it was.

As it turns out, the study was funded by the National Confectioners Association, the trade group that represents all the major candy manufacturers. And the study's findings were actually so weak that one of its coauthors privately called them "thin and clearly padded." Even the study report itself cautioned that "cause and effect associations cannot be drawn," but the candy trade group's press release made no mention of this ginormous disclaimer—if you can call a statement that basically guts the entire study a "disclaimer." Instead, this crazily counterintuitive finding—candy prevents weight gain in kids!—became irresistible Internet click-bait.

Food and beverage companies frequently fund studies like these in hopes of finding the slightest nutritional benefit to tout in their product marketing. And as long as such studies are carried out by independent researchers, this practice shouldn't be a problem. But whether due to researchers' unconscious (or perhaps even conscious) desire to please their benefactors, or because companies inappropriately meddle with the study design, it's now well documented that industry-sponsored studies almost always yield findings that benefit the industry.

Here are a few more examples, among many: a study claiming that oatmeal is more filling than cold cereal, funded by Quaker Oats; a study linking chickpeas to better nutrient intake, funded by Sabra, a maker of chickpea hummus; and a study linking Concord grape juice to improved cognitive function, funded by Welch's. Similarly, in 2018, researchers reviewed fifteen years' worth of studies looking at a possible link between soda consumption and weight gain and diabetes. Of the thirty-four studies that confirmed the link, only one of them had ties to the beverage industry. Of the twenty-six studies that found no such link, every single one of them had industry ties.

This list goes on and on. In fact, when Marion Nestle, an emeritus professor of nutrition and food studies at New York University, kept a running score of all the industry-sponsored studies that came across her desk in 2015, she found that of the 168 studies she reviewed, an astonishing 90 percent had yielded findings favorable to their corporate sponsors. This was true even when other, independently sponsored research looked at the same questions and came to the opposite conclusions.

Another way in which the industry at least arguably attempts to shape scientific debate is by making significant financial contributions to leading health and medical associations. Coca-Cola, for example, has given millions of dollars to organizations like the American Academy of Pediatrics, the American College of Cardiology, the American Academy of Family Physicians, and the American Cancer Society, as well as sponsoring some of their conferences. Coca-Cola also provided millions to the Global Energy Balance Network, a nonprofit led by scientists whose research focused solely on the role of exercise in obesity, ignoring the contribution of sugary beverage consumption. When the *New York Times* exposed Coke's role in funding that organization, it soon disbanded.

### Studies (the Ones We Didn't Pay for) Are "Junk Science"!

Long before every pack of cigarettes came with a warning label, the tobacco industry realized its best defense against lawsuits and governmental regulation was to sow doubt in the minds of the public about the documented harms of smoking. Today, the food and beverage industries use this same playbook: When a well-designed, peer-reviewed study makes the case against consuming a particular food or beverage, industry spokespeople will still call it "junk science," or they'll airily dismiss large bodies of evidence as "inconclusive" or "not definitive"—even when that's not remotely the case.

As just one example, when a governmental committee recommended in 2015 that Americans cut back on sugar—hardly controversial advice— the food and beverage industries went on high alert, retaining no fewer than twenty paid experts to tell the media there was "conflicting science" surrounding the issue. And when we consumers hear those buzzwords repeatedly in the media, we're left believing nothing is yet "settled" scientifically about a given food or beverage, even when it actually is.

### A Trustworthy "Institute" (That We Happen to Fund) Says Our Products Are Just Fine!

The International Life Sciences Institute. The American Council on Science and Health. The International Food Information Council.

All of these groups sound like trustworthy, objective sources of information, right? But in reality, they (and many more like them) are funded by food and beverage companies to allow the industry to engage in so-called "information laundering": hiding behind seemingly neutral organizations to get pro-industry talking points into the media, without having its obviously profit-motivated fingerprints all over the effort.

Companies also create their own "research institutes," like Coke's Beverage Institute for Health and Wellness, or the Gatorade Sports Science Institute, which are staffed by doctors, researchers, and PR professionals ready to offer a unified counter-message to the media on any scientific findings that might harm the company's bottom line. But most of us are entirely unaware of the millions of dollars being spent in these ways to keep us guessing about who's actually telling the truth.

### It's Dietitian Approved! (Just Don't Look at Who's Paying the Dietitian!)

Is a small can of soda a "healthy" snack, analogous to a pack of almonds? It is when the registered dietitian offering that nutritional advice just happens to be paid by Coca-Cola.

For decades, the food and beverage industries have done all they can to cozy up to the Academy of Nutrition and Dietetics, the country's largest organization of registered dietitians. In the past, companies paid sizable fees to sponsor the academy's annual conferences, used their own paid scientists to provide continuing education sessions for dietitians, and flooded its conference expos with massive booths promoting the very types of foods and drinks any responsible dietitian would tell clients to avoid.

Thanks to a reform-minded group called Dietitians for Professional Integrity, the worst of these practices have been curbed in recent years, though not entirely eliminated. But individual nutrition professionals still routinely partner with brands, and while most choose to promote only healthy products, that's not always the case. For example, in 2015 I went head-to-head with McDonald's (in an advocacy campaign I'll tell you about in Chapter 8), and was surprised to find myself sparring on national television with a paid McDonald's "nutritional consultant," one of a whole team of registered dietitians retained by the company to boost its beleaguered image in the media.

And dietitians aren't the only people taking money from the food and beverage industries in exchange for their influence. "Mom bloggers" and popular mom Instagrammers are also aggressively courted, usually with free samples but sometimes with outright payments, in hopes of garnering a favorable post or tweet that will reach their huge followings. This practice is legal as long as the influencers disclose the compensation, but there's no single prescribed way of doing so. Bloggers typically use clear disclosures at the beginning or end of their posts, but on more space-limited platforms like Twitter and Instagram, influencers typically rely on short hashtags like #ad or #sp (signifying "sponsored post") that are easily overlooked if they appear—as they often do—in a dense sea of other hashtags.

McDonald's is worth mentioning again, since it sought out mom influencers from the earliest days of blogging. The company has sponsored women-only blogging conferences like BlogHer (including throwing "Cheeseburg Her" parties for attendees), held "listening tours" for moms, and has even flown select bloggers to its headquarters, all expenses paid. The result of this concerted mom-wooing includes glowing blog posts like "5 Reasons Why Your Family Needs to Visit McDonald's," written by paid "ambassadors," as well as artfully staged Instagram photos showing the kids of popular influencers eating Happy Meals. All of this seemingly spontaneous coverage from trusted moms lends a healthier, more acceptable gloss to the company's mostly unhealthy food.

And remember those Gerber Organic Farm Greens Veggie Crisps I mentioned earlier? A quick Google search led me to a popular mom blogger—compensated by Gerber—who wrote enthusiastically about how "healthy" the snacks are for her picky toddler. But under federal regulations, this product can't use the term "healthy" on its packaging. The blogger stated that the post's content was her own, which I don't doubt, but nonetheless a paid-for post with a misleading "healthy" message still slipped through to her many followers.

Mom influencers are also sometimes co-opted by the industry on matters of scientific debate. In 2014, the chemical company Monsanto paid mom bloggers $150 to sit through a Monsanto-friendly, three-hour informational brunch on "food and farming." A few years earlier, the Corn Refiners Association—makers of high fructose corn syrup—offered $50 Walmart gift cards to induce mom bloggers to listen to a series of presentations by paid scientific experts hoping to increase moms' acceptance of the much-maligned sweetener. And while attendees at these events weren't required to write favorable posts afterward, many did—even if they lacked the expertise to sort fact from fiction in these PR-driven "educational" programs.

## A Case Study: The "Kid/Mom Dynamic"

In 2010, the food giant ConAgra had a problem on its hands. The company's Kid Cuisine frozen meals had long been, in the words of its marketing agency, a "kid-driven request item," meaning children would beg their parents to buy them. And no wonder: the brand's many nutritionally questionable combos looked like they'd been designed by a panel of hopped-up fourth graders: cheeseburgers or mac and cheese served with corn and gummy candy, chicken nuggets served with French fries and pudding, and so on.

But by 2010, the childhood obesity epidemic was very much in the news. Moms were now "less sure of whether they could feel good about serving" Kid Cuisine, according to the company's marketers, and these concerns were becoming a "barrier to more frequent purchase." So ConAgra's marketing agency, the Geppetto Group, turned to its proprietary "Kid/Mom Dynamic" model to figure out the best approach to reboot the brand's image.

Geppetto uses a line graph (a close facsimile of which is reproduced below) to illustrate the Kid/Mom Dynamic, asking its clients, "Is your brand optimally positioned between Kid and Mom?"

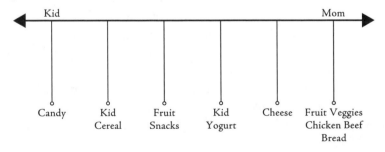

And in this way, Geppetto perfectly—if inadvertently—sums up everything we've just been talking about. Most parents know for sure that foods listed on the "Mom" side of the spectrum are healthy and that candy isn't. But thanks to an incredibly well-funded, concerted, and often covert industry effort to sow confusion, they often feel hopelessly lost within that huge mushy middle. Is "kid yogurt" OK for my child if it contains a ton of sugar but also provides calcium? Can I put any stock in the "contains vitamin C" claim on a box of "fruit snacks"? My child's favorite "kid cereal" looks like an awful lot like junk food, but it's a "good source of whole grains"—so do I buy it or not?

You won't be surprised to hear how the Geppetto Group eventually solved ConAgra's problem. Consistent with Dan Parker's observation, the marketers homed in on that same key question: "What's in it for Mum?" And after concluding that "[m]oms just needed to be informed that Kid Cuisine was a whole lot better than they thought," the agency then came up with the slogan, "The more you know, the less you 'no,'" which they blasted out through print ads, television commercials, a new informational website, and "blogger outreach."

The whole idea behind the campaign was to give moms more "good reasons" to "say yes" to Kid Cuisine. But as with so many of the nutritionism-style pitches discussed here, the "good reasons" were pretty anemic upon closer examination. They mostly relied on minor nutritional tweaks, like the fact that the fried nuggets were breaded with whole grain flour, or assurances that "many" or "most" (but not all) Kid Cuisine meals offered various vitamins and other nutrients.

So even as it encouraged moms to say "yes" to Kid Cuisine, Geppetto also did everything in its power to get kids to pester their moms for the product in the first place. It advised ConAgra to create a new line of special, limited edition "Kombo" meals, which mixed two different themes (like "rock stars" and "dinosaurs") because its market research had shown that "our core target dug the fantasy of mashing two incongruous evergreen themes together." The agency also overhauled the design of the Kid Cuisine cartoon penguin mascot, created a "Krazy Kombo" television commercial targeted directly at children, and came up with a daily instant-win game through which kids were awarded a host of "Krazy Kombo" prizes and a chance to win $1,000 in "Krazy Kombo Ka$h."

Geppetto's "dual targeted" strategy paid off for ConAgra in spades. Within just seventeen days, over 20,000 kids signed up online to play the game, which in the end was played almost 600,000 times. Even better, Geppetto's research showed that kids were coming back again and again to get another crack at winning. Once there, they were also "sticking around to play branded games," each time spending an average of seventeen minutes doing so—a lifetime in terms of targeted advertising exposure.

And writ large, this is how the entire industry operates: divide and conquer the family unit by doing everything allowed by law to erode parents' nutritional vigilance, while doing everything allowed by law to stoke kids' demands for unhealthy products. But what happens when children become dehumanized in this way—when an immensely powerful, well-funded industry sees them not as vulnerable humans with developing bodies and minds, but instead as a "core target" in the never-ending quest for market share?

The short answer: they don't stand a chance.

# 4

# PESTER POWER

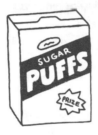

*We don't have TV, but somehow my child comes home*
*from school asking for Froot Loops. He even knows the bird's name is Sam.*

~ MOM OF TWO, KATY, TEXAS

There are certain time-honored truths about parenting. Only after your preschooler is combed, dressed, and buckled into her car seat will she suddenly need to pee. The probability of a toddler meltdown is directly proportional to the number of judgmental bystanders around to witness it. And if you grocery shop with your kids, expect at least six junky products to "magically appear" in your cart before you make it to the checkout lane.

That last one is actually backed up by a study finding that children put an average of six items in their parent's cart during a given grocery outing. Not surprisingly, there's also research showing that snack foods, sweets, and sugary cereals inspire the most nagging. Studies have also found that kids beg for a desired product an average of nine times before a parent caves; the more familiar a child is with popular cartoon characters, the more likely she is to whine for products in the grocery store; and all of this nagging is seriously frustrating for moms and dads.

At the same time, though, most parents are so used to being pestered, they just accept this battle of wills as the natural order of things: kids are hardwired to beg for junk food, embattled parents try to hold the line, and the last one standing determines which products make it home. Yet this dynamic is anything but natural. Believe it or not, there was once a time when companies selling children's products targeted *parents* with their advertising, not kids. Adults controlled the purse strings, after all, and children were supposed to be "seen and not heard," so there was little point in trying to stoke kids' desires.

All of that changed with the dawn of "Pester Power," the ad industry's term for kids' ability to get parents to buy something they (*really, really*) want. Some observers date its origins to 1952, when the first-ever toy commercial, for Mr. Potato Head, ran on television. But according to social historian Lisa Jacobson, marketers started to capitalize on kids' nagging a lot earlier—in the late nineteenth and early twentieth centuries. That's when the publishing industry began to reach kids through popular youth magazines like *Boy's Life, American Girl,* and *Youth's Companion,* and children also started to have more say in family life. Suddenly advertisers had both the motive and the means to exploit kids' new power over the family purse.

Once they saw the profitability of Pester Power, advertisers could hardly contain their enthusiasm. A 1933 printing trade journal article—literally titled "Advertising to the Child to Reach the Parents"—observed: "To use good old circus parlance, every parent is a sucker when it comes to children." A 1919 children's magazine assured potential advertisers that kids "have a way of…getting what they set their hearts on," while an advertising expert advised in 1931 that kids are "bait with which to catch the adult consumer." And in a particularly quaint description of Pester Power, a 1938 advertising journal asked, "[W]ho can long resist the appeal of a child filled with great desire?"

Who indeed? Turning kids into little salesmen proved so successful that some advertisers even coached kids on how to close the deal. Jacobson describes a 1930 ad for roller skates, for example, which urged girls to "[t]ell Daddy and Mother" that the skates would "build sturdy bodies and stronger ankles." A 1916 ad for a bike accessory (with the headline "Please—Father—Please") suggested that boys tell their dads they needed the product so they "could run errands for Mother ever so quick," while a 1932 ad consisted of a comic strip called "How Tom Got His Train." (Spoiler: by lighting Dad's cigarette and generally buttering him up.) Girls might be instructed to take a more coquettish approach, as in an ad suggesting they "whisper to Dad" that Mother needs a new watch (allowing her daughter to wear the old one) "because she's the nicest person in the world...except maybe you."

These days, food and beverage companies are far too savvy to openly refer to kids as "bait," and the majority also adhere to voluntary advertising guidelines forbidding marketers from expressly urging kids to nag their parents. These guidelines, created by the Council of Better Business Bureaus, also state that ads should influence the parent-child relationship only "in a constructive manner."

But every now and then, an advertising executive will slip up and publicly admit it's still all about Pester Power:

+ *"Children are much easier to reach with advertising. They pick up on it fast and quite often we can exploit that relationship and get them pestering their parents."*—an executive at the global ad agency, Saatchi & Saatchi.

+ *"Somebody asked me, 'Lucy, is that ethical? You're essentially manipulating these children.' Well, yeah, is it ethical? I don't know. But our role...is to move product. And we know if we move product...then we've done our job."*—a marketing executive speaking about a study called "The Nag Factor," commissioned to help companies more effectively stoke kids' pestering.

+ *"All our advertising is targeted to kids. You want that nag factor so that seven-year-old Sarah is nagging Mom in the grocery store to buy Funky Purple [a new purple ketchup for kids]. We're not sure Mom would reach out for it on her own."*—a senior brand manager at Heinz.

In fact, almost every "Pretty please, Mom?" heard in the grocery store is the product of an industry effort that's "predetermined, calculated, and analyzed to the nth degree," says Dan Parker, the former British marketer for Big Food. "Nothing is by chance. And I've never met anybody who worked for these companies who wasn't extraordinarily bright and hard-working and ambitious, and with resources that most other organizations can only dream of."

Why are food and beverage companies so determined to reach kids? For one thing, Pester Power is remarkably potent: children under twelve reportedly influence $500 billion in household purchases each year. Today's kids also control a surprising amount of their own money: Children aged three to eleven collectively spend around $40 billion a year, while teens spend almost $160 billion. (Someone out there is clearly giving their kids a really great allowance.) But most important, research shows that brand preferences formed in childhood tend to last a lifetime. As one marketing report recently advised, companies should try to "capture" kids before the age of six, because that's when "brand loyalty begins."

All of this explains why a company selling toaster pastries is desperate to reach kids barely old enough to operate a toaster. Even so, the scale of the industry's efforts is still astonishing.

### A Massive War Chest

Blanketing kids with marketing messages doesn't come cheap. The food and beverage industries won't publicly reveal their advertising budgets, but when the Federal Trade Commission subpoenaed this information in 2009, it discovered that these two industries had collectively spent $1.8 billion that year to market their brands *just* to children.

To put that nearly $2 billion figure in perspective: They'd spent almost a quarter of a million dollars *every single hour of every single day for an entire year* to reach children's eyes and ears. Or as Dr. Kelly Brownell, director of the World Food Policy Center at Duke University's Sanford School of Public Policy, observed in 2012: "[T]he Robert Wood Johnson Foundation is now by far the largest funder of work in this country on childhood obesity. They're spending $100 million a year on the problem. The food industry spends that amount [on child-directed marketing] by January 4th."

And there's no reason to think these industries are spending any less today. If anything, they may be getting even more bang for their buck, thanks to newer and cheaper digital marketing platforms.

## The Latest Brain Science

To better crack kids' psyches and make sure their ads hit home, many brands also consult with experts in child brain development and child psychology.

A pioneer in this questionable merger of science and commerce was Dr. Dan Acuff, a psychologist who ran his own youth marketing firm and also wrote a widely read 1997 book called *What Kids Buy and Why: The Psychology of Marketing to Kids*. Acuff's co-contributor, Dr. Robert Reiher, is an expert in neuroscience and consciousness, and together they meticulously broke down every stage of children's cognitive and emotional development to help advertisers better stimulate kids' desire for their products.

If nothing else, the book is remarkable for its shamelessness, including—I kid you not—advice on how to reach the "birth-to-two-year-old" set. (Sample tip: prey on toddlers' high need for love and security through promotions using softly rounded animal characters with no visible teeth.) But within a few years, even Reiher felt some qualms about the publication of *What Kids Buy and Why*. According to Juliet Schor, a Boston College sociology professor who interviewed him in the early 2000s, Reiher reportedly regretted sharing his research and said he was "disappointed by his experiences in the field of children's marketing. He had hoped to get across a message about the potential misuse of brain science, and to encourage more ethical behavior by marketers." Instead, he told Schor, he "felt that his discussions fell on deaf ears and that for the most part, marketers were interested in using brain science and media psychology to sell more stuff." Shocking.

But Acuff and Reiher weren't alone in peddling their scientific expertise to companies. The ad agency Saatchi & Saatchi once hired a team of clinical psychologists and cultural anthropologists to spend more than five hundred hours observing and interviewing children to better understand how to market to them online. By 1999, so many child psychologists were doing this kind of work that sixty of their disgusted colleagues sent an open letter to the American Psychological Association denouncing the practice as "abuse" and a "crisis for the profession." They also urged the organization to "establish limits... regarding the use of psychological knowledge or techniques to observe, study, manipulate, harm, exploit, mislead, trick or deceive children for commercial purpose."

The organization never established those limits, and today's youth marketing firms still promise, for example, that their expertise in "kids, developmental psychology and neuroscience" will offer clients "new tools and pathways" to reach children. In a testimonial, another such firm's pleased client said its marketers had the "knowledge of a development psych professor" which they used to "translate genuine child development insights into business-growing ideas."

### Et Tu, Dora?

To target the youngest kids, one of the most potent weapons in the marketer's arsenal is the cartoon character, whether licensed from television and movies, like Dora the Explorer, or specially created for a brand, like Tony the Tiger. These beloved fictional friends are especially valuable when used on product packaging and in-store displays, where they're virtually guaranteed to catch kids' eyes in the grocery store.

"It's all about forming a relationship with a child," explains Dr. Marlene Schwartz, director of the Rudd Center for Food Policy & Obesity at the University of Connecticut. "The child already feels an affinity toward SpongeBob or Dora, and you're connecting that relationship with the food product." One leading researcher has even said that, once forged, this emotional connection "is basically impossible to get rid of." Indeed, just seeing a familiar character on a product actually causes children to prefer the food's taste over the same food packaged without it, an effect that's unfortunately stronger for junk food than for healthy food.

When parents first see this phenomenon in action, they often can't believe how powerful it is. A mother of a three-year-old told a researcher, "She is [just becoming] aware of more characters. [She] doesn't know what the product is but she wants it. I'm shocked by her awareness.... She'll have full-on tantrums.... it's amazing." Another mom, one who strictly limits her five-year-old's screen viewing, still reported, "She picks up on characters almost by osmosis. I avoid ads, but she still notices, and [the ads] are manipulative."

This use of characters is such a blatant exploitation of young children's emotions that even Acuff and Reiher, the authors of *What Kids Buy and Why*, recognized in a later book that, depending on the nature of the advertised product, it had "a potential for harming the child's emotional, physical, or psychological development." Using Joe Camel to sell cigarettes "must not be allowed," they wrote, yet they deemed character marketing for unhealthy food a "neutral" practice, albeit one that was "acceptable only in limited or controlled amounts."

Notably, though, they didn't direct those words of caution toward the food-industry clients funding their work. Instead, they wrote, "[P]arents might occasionally yield to their children's request for a sugary cereal promoted by [a character] but the parents should do so only rarely." In other words: Sure, it's irresponsible, but it's still your problem, not ours.

## Seriously, Shaquille?

Children eventually outgrow their love of cartoon characters, but marketers are no less willing to capitalize on older kids' adoration for famous athletes, film stars, and musicians. Yet the companies most able to pay multimillion dollar endorsement fees also tend to make the least healthy products. When a 2016 study looked at the products associated with kids' favorite music stars—including Beyoncé, Usher, and Britney Spears—it found that 71 percent of the promoted drinks were sugary, and more than 80 percent of the foods were unhealthy.

And even though most star athletes presumably eat healthfully in private, they, too, seem to have no qualms about promoting junk food. Venus and Serena Williams were paid to endorse Triple Stuff Oreos, as were Eli and Peyton Manning, Apollo Ohno, and Shaquille O'Neal. Peyton Manning also hawked Papa John's Pizza; O'Neal pitched Burger King; and early in his career, LeBron James was a front man for McDonald's. Professional sports leagues are no better: a 2018 study found that 76 percent of the products endorsed by leagues like the NFL, NBA, and NHL were unhealthy. Not only do kids draw damaging messages about diet from these paid sports heroes, one study found that even parents mistakenly believe a product is healthier when it's endorsed by an athlete.

## Immersive, Interactive, and Insidious

In 2000, when brands like Kellogg's were launching their first websites, the *New York Times* marveled over the fact that Tony the Tiger was "no longer a still life on a box or a fleeting image on the television screen, but a character, even a friend." Experts quoted in the piece were worried that this (now laughably primitive) interactivity would harm kids, yet today, only the youngest children find much appeal in sitting at their parent's computer to play tame "advergames" with the Lucky Charms leprechaun.

These days, it's all about getting kids to deeply engage with a brand through their mobile devices, using social media platforms like YouTube, Instagram, and Snapchat. And with good reason: a 2018 survey found that 95 percent of teens own a smartphone, with 45 percent reporting they're online "almost constantly" and another 44 percent saying they go online at least several times a day. Younger kids are only somewhat less connected. The vast majority of children under age eight live in homes with a smartphone and an Internet connection, and nearly half of these children already own their own tablet device.

Reaching kids through digital and social media is appealing to food and beverage companies for three reasons: it's cheaper than traditional advertising; kids spend more time interacting with the brand; and it conveniently cuts parents out of the loop. As the Rudd Center's Schwartz puts it, "Most parents have no idea how much their children are being marketed to online."

What does this new digital marketing look like? It's often downright creepy. Here are just some of the ways unhealthy food and drink brands currently "reach out" to children:

+ A student says on Twitter that she has "two finals down, two to go." Minutes later, she receives a friendly tweet from Red Bull, the caffeinated, sugary drink brand, that reads, "Need a study buddy to finish finals season strong?"
+ A thirteen-year-old boy playing the popular NBA2K basketball video game is encouraged to score endorsement contracts for his

virtual NBA player from unhealthy brands like Gatorade, Mountain Dew, and Reese's Puffs. He can also have his player work out in a Gatorade-branded fitness center and earn valuable "energy" by consuming the brand's real-world drinks and energy bars.

+ A boy who is a popular YouTube "influencer" posts a video in which he and his little sister conduct a blind taste test of twenty-five kinds of Pringles. The video garners 37 million views, leading other kids to join in the "Pringles Challenge" with their own videos.

+ A ten-year-old boy plays a Gatorade-sponsored game on his mobile phone in which he's told that water, unlike sugar-sweetened Gatorade, is the "enemy" of athletic performance. (Yes, you read that right.) He has to shoot down drops of water to win the game.

+ A middle schooler uses a special Snapchat lens that turns her face into a giant Taco Bell taco. By the end of the day, the lens will have garnered 224 million views and the average user will have played with the ad for 24 seconds before sending it as a snap.

This is just a small sampling of the kinds of digital promotions currently targeting kids, and marketers' methods are only growing more sophisticated. Also keep in mind that digital marketing can often be specifically tailored to a child's demographics, purchasing data, and even her physical location. Another troubling thought: once a child is pegged as a lover of junk food from his clicking and purchasing history, he may start to see only ads for other unhealthy products, creating a harmful feedback loop.

### We've Got You Surrounded

Digital media may be at the cutting edge of kid-directed junk food marketing, but don't think for a minute that companies have abandoned their old-school methods.

+ Television commercials remain the gold standard for reaching large numbers of children, especially when they're not already familiar with the brand. So today's kids still see about ten to eleven food-related commercials a day, or around four thousand each year.

+ In school, kids may encounter in the cafeteria products bearing junk food brand names like Frosted Flakes and Doritos, be given Pizza Hut reading coupons in class, or learn to count from an Oreo-branded counting book. They might attend school fundraisers like McDonald's "McTeacher's Nights" or be encouraged collect Box Tops, which appear mostly on unhealthy products. McDonald's even tried to get its own branded "nutrition education" film into school classrooms, a campaign I discuss in Chapter 8.

+ Even kids' extracurricular activities aren't safe from marketers' reach. Gatorade helpfully offers young athletes "hydration education," while Little League's sponsors include Frosted Flakes, Gatorade, and Bomb Pops, a brand of sugar-sweetened frozen ice pops.

+ Unhealthy food and beverage marketing creeps into children's lives in more subtle ways, too, like branded toys, corporate sponsorships of events for families and kids, and product placements in popular TV shows and movies.

Put it all together and you have what one child-marketing specialist approvingly calls "surround marketing." Or, as another youth marketer advised her clients, "It isn't enough to just advertise on television. You've got to reach kids throughout their day—in school, as they're shopping at the mall, [and at] the movies. You've got to become part of the fabric of their lives."

*Harming Kids While Undermining Parents*

Not that we needed it, but research confirms that marketing does significantly increase a child's desire for the advertised product. (Why else would these industries pay billions for it?) The American Psychological Association has also found that this desire can be instilled with as little as *one* commercial exposure.

What makes those two findings especially troubling is that the products most heavily marketed to kids are also the ones most harmful to their health. In 2016, kids saw, on average, around eleven TV ads a day for foods and beverages; of these, the overwhelming majority were for fast food, candy, sweet and salty snacks, and sugary drinks, while fewer than 10 percent advertised healthier foods like yogurt, water, or fruits and vegetables. And kids of color get a double dose of this unhealthy food marketing because many food and beverage companies disproportionately target Hispanic and African American children.

If this weren't bad enough, food advertising actually causes children to eat more in the short term. This phenomenon, called "priming," was demonstrated in a 2009 study (among many others) in which kids were given bowls of Goldfish crackers, then left alone to watch a short cartoon containing commercials either for non-food products like games and toys, or for food products commonly advertised on children's television, like sweet cereals and fruit snacks. Those who saw food ads ate 45 percent more Goldfish than kids who'd seen non-food ads. Similarly, a 2018 study in the UK found that when kids saw Instagram posts of popular celebrities enjoying junk food, they later selected less healthy snacks and consumed 26 percent more calories than those in the control group. In fact, a 2015 analysis of forty-five different priming studies not only found that food ads make people eat more, the food cravings they trigger are just as intense as those caused by seeing real food, and even more intense than those caused by smelling enticing food aromas.

Child-directed food and beverage marketing also causes a more insidious harm: the way Pester Power undermines parents' authority and damages their relationship with their kids. Skeptics might scoff at this notion, arguing that parents just need to grow a spine and say "no." But the reality is that parents *do* say "no"—over and over again. When researchers from Johns Hopkins surveyed mothers of young kids in 2011, they found that moms collectively resorted to ten different strategies to deal with nagging. And while most parents know they shouldn't cave, it's not easy to hold the line day in and day out—especially since nagging usually takes place in public, where parents understandably want to avoid conflict.

But whether parents give in or stand firm, all this nagging takes a toll. Surveyed moms used words like "battle," "losses," and "overwhelming" to describe these interactions with their kids, and some admitted they frequently raise their voices and lose their temper. Ultimately, the Johns Hopkins researchers concluded that Pester Power causes a "high level of frustration and stress" for parents and seriously undermines their ability to act as responsible nutritional gatekeepers. And that finding doesn't take into account the *other* major way marketers undermine parents' nutritional gatekeeping: the use of misleading nutrition claims to keep parents in a state of constant confusion.

What's perhaps most sinister about unhealthy food marketing is the way it preys upon kids' immature brain development. Research shows that children under age four or five can't distinguish commercials from programmed content; it's all one big blur of entertainment. And even when kids do start to make that distinction, they still don't understand advertising's purpose, instead viewing it as just another facet of the viewing experience. This cognitive deficit makes kids under age eight sitting ducks for marketers, in that they unquestioningly soak up any messages advertisers want to impart. For that reason, both the American Psychological Association and the American Academy of Pediatrics have stated that marketing anything to children in this age group is inherently unfair and deceptive.

Older children are vulnerable, too. By age nine or ten, kids may generally understand the concept of marketing, but many still don't grasp that an advertiser might want to induce people to buy something they might not otherwise want; one study found only 40 percent of kids aged eleven to twelve truly understood that the advertiser was trying to persuade viewers. And when the line between advertising and content is intentionally blurred, even teenagers may not realize they're being marketed to. That's especially true of more subtle marketing, like the product placements woven into video games, movies, and social media posts by paid celebrities or other influencers on Instagram, Twitter, or YouTube.

If we substituted "tobacco," for "unhealthy foods and drinks" in this chapter, most parents would be outraged at this relentless, profit-driven assault on their kids. And in fact, a 2015 Rudd Center survey found that 85 percent of parents believed food companies should reduce unhealthy food marketing to kids, while 71 percent agreed that food companies act irresponsibly when they advertise to children.

So why hasn't our government tried to rein in the food and beverage industries? The short answer is: It has. *Twice*. And... let's just say, it didn't go very well.

## Kid Vid

Few young parents today are likely aware that in the late 1970s, the Federal Trade Commission (FTC) actually proposed restricting or even banning television commercials directed at children. This regulatory effort, which came to be known as Kid Vid, was motivated by two developments: an alarming rise in kids' dental cavities, at least partially due to all the sugary cereals being advertised on children's television; and then-new research indicating that young kids don't grasp advertising's persuasive intent.

On the basis of that emerging research alone, the FTC concluded that child-directed marketing was unfair and ought to be regulated. And the FTC's then-chairman, Michael Pertschuk, assumed public opinion was on his side. A 1979 ABC News poll found that 79 percent of the public supported a ban on advertising sugary products to kids, while 72 percent supported a ban on all advertising to kids under age eight. As Pertschuk later recalled, he just couldn't imagine "prudent senators and congressmen...enlisting on the...side of 'junk food' advertisers against the health and well-being of the American child and family."

But Pertschuk seriously underestimated Kid Vid's opponents. Together, the major industries that profited from marketing to kids—toy manufacturers, ad agencies, the three national TV networks, and the food and beverage industries—raised $16 million to fight back against the proposed regulation. (That sum may sound paltry today, but back then it represented one-fourth of the FTC's entire operating budget.) The group also proved masterful at reframing the debate: Instead of American families being *protected* by Kid Vid, as the FTC viewed it, these industries accused the agency of acting as a "national nanny" trampling on families' freedom and autonomy.

Pertschuk at first didn't think this "nanny state" messaging would gain much traction. As he later wrote, the entire Kid Vid effort began only after the FTC received numerous "petitions and pleadings" from concerned "parents, teachers, pediatricians, dentists, and others representing mainstream organizations concerned with family health and welfare." But even the usually liberal *Washington Post* eventually adopted the "nanny" narrative in a scathing editorial, mocking the effort as one "designed to protect children from the weaknesses of their parents" instead of from predatory marketing. As Pertschuk later recalled, "[O]nce the issue was framed in these terms, there was no way we could win."

But the FTC didn't just lose out on Kid Vid. It also suffered a permanent blow to its enforcement powers. That's because this all took place at the dawn of the anti-government, pro-business Reagan era, and the backlash against the FTC was particularly fierce. Not only did Congress defund the FTC (a common tactic now, but virtually unheard-of back then), it also stripped the agency of its ability to go after children's advertising on the ground that it's per se unfair to kids. To this day, the FTC first has to prove the advertising is also deceptive—a much higher bar.

It was such a crushing defeat for the agency that even decades later, the mere mention Kid Vid would, in the words of an FTC official speaking in 2004, "send a shudder" through staff members who worked on the effort. No matter how solid a case might be made for banning junk food advertising to children, he said, "[t]he Federal Trade Commission has traveled down this road before. It is not a journey that anyone at the commission cares to repeat."

### Letting the Fox Guard the Henhouse

Kid Vid may have killed the federal government's appetite for regulating children's advertising, but a public health crisis far more serious than dental cavities—rising childhood obesity—forced it to reconsider in 2005.

That's when the Institute of Medicine (IOM, now the National Academy of Medicine—the nonprofit that advises the federal government on matters related to health and medicine) warned Congress that "urgent preventive actions" were needed to halt kids' rising weight gain. The report also specifically cited child-directed food and beverage advertising as likely playing a role in the crisis. Congress asked the IOM to study the question in greater depth, and a year later the IOM released a report confirming that this marketing did in fact cause "children to prefer and request high-calorie and low-nutrient foods and beverages" while contributing to "an environment that puts their health at risk." The IOM's report therefore urged the food and beverage industries to clean up their act, adding ominously that if they didn't, "Congress should enact legislation."

So in 2007, a group of leading food and beverage companies got together and did what industries often do when threatened with government oversight: they formed a self-regulatory program. Today, eighteen major industry players are members of the Children's Food and Beverage Advertising Initiative (CFBAI), which is dedicated to voluntarily improving child-directed food and drink advertising. These companies generate the vast majority of this advertising, and as part of their membership, each has pledged to: only market "healthier dietary choices" to kids under twelve; not use licensed characters to market unhealthy foods to kids; and stay out of elementary schools.

But if you're having trouble squaring those benevolent promises with your child's daily reality, you're not alone. The disconnect, predictably, can be explained by the fine print of the CFBAI pledge, which has so many loopholes it's like a piece of (highly processed, artificially colored and flavored) Swiss cheese.

The biggest loophole relates to which products qualify as "healthier dietary choices" that can still be freely advertised to kids. For the first six years of the program, each CFBAI member was actually allowed to create its own nutritional guidelines, resulting in an approved product list that included items like Lucky Charms, Froot Loops, and Fruity Pebbles cereals; Pepperoni Pizza Lunchables; Kool-Aid Singles drink mix; Baked Cheetos cheese puffs; and Gushers fruit snacks. (After seeing a list of these products in a focus group, one dismayed parent asked, "If these are the better-for-you foods, what's the worst list?")

The industry pledge also only applies to advertising on "child-directed" media, which the CFBAI currently defines as media for which children make up at least 35 percent of the audience.* This means Saturday morning cartoons and other clearly kid-centric shows are off- limits, but many

---

* In the early years of the program, each CFBAI member was allowed to set its own criteria for what constituted "child-directed media," and some companies set an even more industry-friendly bar, such as requiring that at least 50 percent of the audience consist of children under twelve.

other programs also regularly watched by millions of young children—like variety shows and "family friendly" sitcoms and dramas—remain open season. And while the CFBAI defines "children" as kids under twelve, many health advocates believe the pledge should extend to children under fifteen due to their continued susceptibility to marketing.

The CFBAI promise to stay out of elementary schools also sounds solid, but if you happen to read the footnotes (pro tip: *always* read the footnotes), you'll see that the program still allows every one of the in-school marketing methods mentioned earlier, like McTeacher's Nights, Box Top collections, branded cafeteria food, and fast-food coupons for classroom achievement.

Another weakness in the program: CFBAI companies can freely advertise their brand to children even if just one product under that brand is a "healthier dietary choice." So, for example, McDonald's can blanket children's television with Happy Meal commercials if the particular meal depicted (often fleetingly) includes apple slices and milk instead of fries and a soda, and Kraft Heinz can hawk Lunchables meals to kids if its ad depicts one of just three varieties that meet CFBAI nutrition standards—out of the over thirty kinds of Lunchables currently sold.

And finally, CFBAI members promise not to use licensed characters or movie tie-ins when marketing less healthy products to kids. But that pledge doesn't include a company's own characters, like Toucan Sam, and—loophole alert!—it also doesn't extend to product packaging, in-store displays, or premium giveaways. Yet these particular uses of licensed characters—think: Happy Meal toys, cereal boxes, cardboard cut-outs in the supermarket—are among *the* most powerful ways to stoke Pester Power.

Two years after the CFBAI was formed, a 2009 study checked in on the program's progress. Given all these glaring loopholes, you won't be surprised to learn that two-thirds of the CFBAI products marketed to kids were still so unhealthy that they fell into the category of foods and drinks the federal government says people should consume only on "special occasions, such as your birthday." Ads for fruits and vegetables accounted for less than one percent of all CFBAI advertising, while the proportion of CFBAI ads featuring licensed characters had nearly doubled, with roughly half of those ads promoting unhealthy foods.

Self-regulation clearly wasn't cutting it, and since Democrats controlled both the White House and Congress when the 2009 CFBAI study was released, the climate seemed ripe for reform. So Congress directed four federal agencies—the FTC, the Food and Drug Administration, the Centers for Disease Control, and the Department of Agriculture—to come up with a stronger set of nutrition standards for marketing foods and drinks to kids. These standards would be purely voluntary (no one was looking for a repeat of Kid Vid), but the hope was that companies would still feel pressured to adopt them.

At first it seemed like this "Interagency Working Group on Food Marketed to Children" (IWG) was off to a solid start. Michelle Obama's Let's Move! Initiative was going strong, and the First Lady had even given a speech to the Grocery Manufacturers Association (the food and beverage industries' trade group) chastising its members for pushing junk food on kids. Alluding to the damning CFBAI study, she said, "[I]n the face of these statistics, we have to ask ourselves, are we really making sufficient progress here? Are we doing everything that we can to secure the health and future of our kids?"

With this increased public scrutiny, food and beverage companies knew they had to do better. They were not, however, going to let a bunch of meddlesome federal agencies tell them how to do it. So when the IWG finally released its proposed guidelines in 2011—by which time, control of the House of Representatives had shifted to Republicans—these two industries were ready for a brawl.

Partnering with entertainment companies like Walt Disney and Viacom (owner of the children's channel Nickelodeon), the food and beverage industries had already formed a front group called the Sensible Food Policy Coalition to undermine the IWG's efforts. The coalition claimed the guidelines would somehow kill 400,000 jobs, result in $152 billion in lost revenue, and prevent the marketing of even healthy foods like yogurt and whole wheat bread. It hired a big-gun constitutional law expert to say that the guidelines—though voluntary—were unconstitutional. And, of course, the lobbying dollars flowed in by the millions to sway key legislators. (To put these lobbying expenditures in perspective, the Center for Science in the Public Interest, a lead supporter of the

IWG, spent around $70,000 on all of its lobbying efforts in 2011; that year, the food and beverage industries reportedly spent the same amount on lobbying *every 13 hours*.)

As the fight raged on, public health advocates eagerly awaited a response from Michelle Obama. Any minute now, she was going to give a powerful speech that would refocus the debate on what really mattered: the health of America's kids. But it turned out they were waiting in vain. Throughout the entire controversy, neither the First Lady nor anyone else from the White House spoke up to defend the IWG's mission.

Months after its opponents in Congress officially killed the IWG, a special Reuters report shed light on what had gone down. An examination of White House visitor logs revealed that, at the height of the IWG fight, a group of major food and entertainment industry players had been granted an audience with top Obama administration officials, including senior advisor Valerie Jarrett. Attendees included executives from Nestlé, Kellogg's, General Mills, Walt Disney, Time Warner, and Viacom, as well as the lead lobbyist for the Grocery Manufacturers Association and the CFBAI's president.

With President Obama's re-election campaign in full swing, the White House likely had no desire to make enemies of these deep-pocketed companies. But whatever the reason, Reuters reported that after that meeting, "the administration stood back at crucial junctures, allowing Congress time to thwart the [IWG] effort." The First Lady also began to shift the focus of Let's Move! from healthy food to increasing physical activity—mirroring the industry's own emphasis on exercise to deflect criticism of its unhealthy products. "I'd focus more on exercise, too, if my husband was up for re-election," Margo Wootan, vice president for nutrition at the Center for Science in the Public Interest, told Reuters.

For public health advocates (and this *Lunch Tray* blogger), it was a heartbreaking betrayal. Even Marion Nestle, the New York University professor who's an expert on food politics, seemed surprised. "It's hard to believe how thoroughly Congress is in bed with the food industry," she wrote. The policy director for Children Now, the group that had commissioned the 2009 study critical of the CFBAI, dejectedly told Reuters, "Money wins." And former Senator Tom Harkin, an original champion of the IWG, criticized the White House for caving in to corporate influence.

"They went wobbly in the knees," he lamented. "When it comes to kids' health, they shouldn't go wobbly in the knees."

Just as with Kid Vid thirty years before, the food and beverage industries triumphed. But to help protect its members from any future threat of regulation, the CFBAI did finally close one of its biggest loopholes. Instead of continuing to allow members to come up with their own lax nutrition standards, the CFBAI formally adopted uniform standards to apply across the board.

I regard these new standards as "slightly-better-than-better-for-you," meaning they do represent an improvement over the earlier standards (how could they not?). But few parents would regard the qualifying products as actually *healthy*. Examples from CFBAI's 2018 approved product list include Frosted Flakes, Lucky Charms, Trix, Fruity Pebbles, Froot Loops, Cookie Crisp, and Reese's Peanut Butter Puffs cereals; Kool-Aid Singles drink mix; Jolly Rancher Popsicles; Flavor Blasted Goldfish crackers; Kid Cuisine Popcorn Chicken frozen meals; and Pepperoni Pizza Lunchables. Perhaps this fact says it all: most of the products CFBAI members are still allowed to market to your kids can't legally be sold in public schools due to their excessive calories, sugar, and/or fat.*

And by the way, in case you're wondering, here's the IWG's own description of what its voluntary guidelines were meant to achieve, if they hadn't been killed by the industry: "Advertising and marketing should encourage children to choose foods that make meaningful contributions to a healthful diet from food groups including vegetables, fruit, whole grains, fat-free or low-fat milk products, fish, extra lean meat and poultry, eggs, nuts or seeds, and beans. In addition, the saturated fat, trans fat, added sugars, and sodium in foods marketed to children should be limited to minimize the negative impact on children's health and weight."

That's it.

Just common sense guidance that would have dramatically improved the children's food and beverage advertising landscape. But that guidance also collided with one hard truth: the processed food industry sells very

---

* To conform with the 2015–2020 Dietary Guidelines for Americans, an updated version of the CFBAI's uniform nutrition standards will go into effect in 2020. But if history is any guide, don't expect major changes to CFBAI's approved product list.

few healthy foods, while earning billions every year selling unhealthy ones. And there was no way it was ever going to accept child marketing guidelines that didn't accommodate that reality.

* * *

In the years since the IWG dust-up, not a whole lot has changed. A 2017 study marking the tenth anniversary of the CFBAI found that, overall, there's been 45 percent reduction in the number of food ads on children's television. That's good news, of course, but at least part of this reduction only reflects the industry's new focus on cheaper digital marketing. In fact, thanks to the CFBAI's relatively narrow definition of what constitutes "child-directed" media, kids are still seeing, on average, three television commercials a day for products from CFBAI members that aren't "better-for-you," along with marketing for such products using all the other channels that fall outside their pledge: product packaging, in-school promotions, YouTube videos, smartphone apps, and more. And since kids older than eleven remain fair game, the 2017 study also found that "[s]ome CFBAI companies appeared to be directly targeting young teens with ads for candy, sugary drinks, snack foods, and fast food."

None of this comes as a surprise to Parker, the former British ad executive, who's fighting his own battle over self-regulation of kids' advertising in the UK. "I find it very hard to live with the idea that you could ask any industry to self-regulate when so much money is at stake," he says. "It's like asking a child to decide what time they go to bed. No child is ever going to say anything acceptable, are they?"

Parker knows from experience that food and beverage companies will only make the concessions least likely to cut into their profits. "But if you say, 'How about don't use children's characters in order to sell junk food?'—on that kind of stuff, they won't even engage in a conversation," Parker says. "Because that's what works."

And yet, according to Parker, many of the individual men and women who work on child-directed junk food campaigns—the account execs, the creative directors, the brand managers—secretly wish the government *would* step in and regulate them. "I find that an awful lot of people who work in advertising actually feel quite vulnerable at the moment," he says, "because they're not comfortable about the work they have to do in order to compete. None of us want to be the Mad Men of cigarette advertising. We don't want to sit there in twenty years' time, and have our children say, 'So, Daddy, what did you do?' 'Well, I sold fizzy drinks to children.' No one wants to be that person."

For now, though, Parker feels marketers are in an impossible bind. "If you turn around and say to Coca-Cola, 'We don't want to go with that idea because we're a bit too uncomfortable with it,' well, you just don't have Coca-Cola as a client anymore, do you?" says Parker, "You don't have a great deal of choice."

So until elected officials are able to resist food and beverage companies' lobbying, exhausted parents will be left on their own to hold the line against Pester Power—even as these two industries continue to spend billions to stoke it. Or as one marketing insider recently put it, "It's the circle of retail life. Child demands product, parent learns about product through child, household begins using product, child ideally grows up to encourage his or her own household to use said product—at least until their own kids start making requests."

As long as there's money to be made, whether "product harms child" is beside the point.

# 5

# CAFETERIA COPYCATS

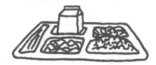

*[My children's cafeteria offers] so many fried foods
or just unhealthy or uninspired choices like hot dogs and hamburgers.
There are way too many bad choices in the à la carte.*

~ MOM OF FOUR, PLYMOUTH MEETING, PA

When I think back to the food served in my elementary school in the early 1970s, what comes to mind is pretty close to the iconic image of an old-fashioned school lunch: a pistachio-green tray filled with spaghetti or meatloaf, along with sides like canned green beans and fruit cocktail. And while some dishes were certainly more popular than others—like the rectangular "pizza" served a few times a month—I don't recall ever feeling actively *courted* by the cafeteria. It was just implicitly understood that students were the passive recipients of whatever food the school chose to provide, some of which we liked and some of which we griped about. And if you had the option of bringing lunch from home—which, in my case, may or may not have been toted in a Partridge Family lunchbox—you consulted the school menu printed weekly in the local newspaper (geez, I really am dating myself) and decided whether you wanted to buy it.

Today, though, that dynamic has been flipped on its head. Children are now seen less as grateful beneficiaries of a hot meal and more like fickle, paying customers who have to be lured into the cafeteria by any means necessary. Just take a look at the kid-enticing, fast-food-style entrées served during a single week in 2018 in the elementary schools of Appling County, Georgia:

- ✦ Chicken Sandwich with Waffle Fries
- ✦ Pepperoni Pizza
- ✦ Hamburger with Seasoned Fries
- ✦ Chicken Tenders with Honey Mustard
- ✦ Hot Dog with Chili and Cheese Tater Tots

The median household income in Appling County is around $30,000—about half the national average—but this type of menu isn't necessarily tied to demographics or socioeconomics. During that same week, the elementary school entrées in Grosse Pointe, Michigan, an affluent Detroit suburb with a median household income of over $100,000, were:

- ✦ Cheese Stuffed Breadsticks
- ✦ Macaroni and Cheese
- ✦ Classic Cheeseburger in Bun
- ✦ Whole Grain French Toast Sticks
- ✦ Cheese or Classic Pepperoni Pizza

For all their economic differences, kids in these two districts—and in so many others around the country—are seeing the same sorts of "carnival food" in their cafeterias on a weekly basis.

As Janet Poppendieck explains in *Free for All: Fixing School Food in America*, the evolution from homestyle to fast-food-style menus began in the mid to late 1970s. This is when kids were first allowed to select just three out of five meal components as they went through the lunch line, a change meant to reduce food waste but one that also gave children a more active role in shaping school meals. The late 1970s and early 1980s also marked a period of severe cuts to federal school meal funding, which sent many districts into the arms of processed food manufacturers (and even fast food chains) promising to do the job on the cheap. Many districts also started selling junk food in their à la carte lines to bring in additional revenue, but then had to make their school meals look more like junk food to compete with those offerings.

Four decades later, these profound shifts are still evident in today's school menus. The majority are dominated by kid-driven carnival food, and even when school nutrition directors offer healthier entrées like salads and stir-fries, they'll still typically offer a fast food-style entrée on the same day to "hedge their bets" with kids. On a recent day in St. Louis's public schools, for example, the Veggie Wrap was forced to duke it out with the Crispy Corn Dog and the Cheesy Beef Nachos. (We can only guess which entrée won out.)

But other school nutrition directors don't even bother with the Veggie Wraps, and instead push carnival food to the limit. Take "Director X," whom I first encountered in an online forum for school food professionals. The forum typically draws from the most dedicated segment of the profession, yet while other members were proudly showing off photos of their new salad bars, Director X crowed about serving a breakfast of pink frosted donuts, followed by a "breakfast for lunch" menu of sugary funnel cakes, deep-fried potatoes, a sausage patty, chocolate milk, and a shrink-wrapped slice of pallid, unripe watermelon. He described that day's menu as a "sweet deal" for his students and favorably likened it to the food offered at a state fair—a bit of a head-scratcher in the context of a child nutrition program.

Director X also sometimes copies brand-name fast food entrées, like setting up a hot dog bar mimicking the one at James Coney Island (a regional fast food chain), which included fixings like bacon, tortilla chips, crinkle-cut French fries, and Funyuns. But Director X isn't alone in trying to recreate real-world fast food in the lunch room. I've read about other directors' attempts to replicate the Big Mac, entrées from Chick-fil-A, and the KFC Famous Bowl. The latter was once named a "Top 10 Worst Fast Food Meal" by *Time* magazine, but when a school nutrition director posted a photo of her KFC Famous Bowl facsimile—deep-fried chicken fingers served on mashed potatoes, topped with corn, gravy, and shredded cheese—it generated only excitement. "I saw the picture and thought it was a KFC ad.... They look awesome!!!!" wrote one impressed colleague, while another asked about the legality of using fast food brand names on her menu. "Are we allowed to say we are serving KFC Famous Bowls or [a] McRib sandwich?" she asked. "I love love love this idea!"

But districts don't even have to struggle to recreate fast food or junk food in their own kitchens, because the food industry is eager to sell them the real thing. Take Domino's Smart Slice pizza, which districts can have delivered hot to their cafeterias by local franchisees. Smart Slice does meet school nutrition regulations, but the pizza looks just like regular Domino's— right down to the prominently branded cardboard boxes and paper sleeves in which it's served to kids. Districts can also redeem points for yet more Domino's branded items like hats, aprons, and point-of-sale signage because, in the words of one pleased nutrition director appearing in a Smart Slice promotional video, "Just the name Domino's sells the product."

As of 2016, Domino's was reportedly providing Smart Slice to over six thousand districts in forty-seven states, figures that are likely significantly higher today. Other chains, including Papa John's and Pizza Hut, also cater to schools. But branded pizza is just the start. Today's kids are regularly offered in their cafeterias a wide variety of school-compliant products bearing the junk food trademarks they know and love, including Pop-Tarts toaster pastries; Lucky Charms, Frosted Flakes, and Apple Jacks cereal; Cheetos, Doritos, and Funyuns snacks; and sweets like Rice Krispies Treats and bright blue Froot by the Foot.

All of this may come as a surprise if you remember the Obama administration's well-publicized school food reform, which was seen as so stringent by some on the far right that Michelle Obama was frequently mocked as a member of the Food Police. How can we square that criticism with school-sanctioned Tostitos and Frosted Flakes?

The Healthy, Hunger-Free Kids Act (HHFKA), championed by the former First Lady and signed into law in 2010, did make school food a lot healthier. Despite some weakening of its nutrition standards by the Trump administration in 2018, the HHFKA placed reasonable limits on school meals' fat, calories, and sodium, and kids now have to take a half-cup serving of either fruit or vegetables at lunch instead of regularly passing up these healthy foods. Schools must also offer a greater variety of produce, including dark leafy greens and red and orange vegetables, and half of the grain foods served (such as breads and pastas) must be "whole-grain rich," meaning they have to contain at least 50 percent whole grains. (Prior to the Trump administration's roll-back, all grain foods had to be whole-grain rich.)

So there's no question that school meals were significantly improved by the new law, a critical development for the 30 million kids who regularly eat those meals, two-thirds of whom are economically disadvantaged. And while critics contend that the HHFKA's healthier nutrition standards have driven kids from the cafeteria and caused an increase in food waste, a comprehensive 2019 study commissioned by the U.S. Department of Agriculture (USDA) soundly refuted both of those claims.

Those are all very important gains, and I don't want to be seen as minimizing the impressive achievement of getting the HHFKA passed— on a bipartisan basis, no less—or discounting the decades-long efforts of public health advocates that made it possible. But I'd also be lying if I told you that America's school food is now exactly where it should be. Here's where there's still room for improvement:

## A (Too-) Sweet Start to the Day

First, despite the HHKFA's new curbs on calories, fat, and sodium, there's still no limit on the amount of added sugar that can be served to kids in school meals.

This omission wasn't an oversight. When the HHFKA was being debated, there was no federal dietary guidance (as there is now) on how much added sugar is too much for children, so there were no official parameters on which to base regulations. And back then, food manufacturers weren't required to disclose added sugars on their products' Nutrition Facts labels (as they will be starting in 2020), so it would have been difficult at any rate for districts to figure out exactly how much added sugar they were serving kids.

Even without a regulatory cap, though, the amount of sugar in school lunch still tends to be reasonable, thanks to the meal's overall calorie limits and other nutritional requirements. It's in the federal School Breakfast Program where things can really go off the rails. That's because the breakfast regulations don't require a protein entrée like eggs, cheese, or meat. So instead, most districts rely heavily on cheaper grain entrées like cereals, muffins, and breakfast pastries, or on yogurt-based entrées like smoothies and granola parfaits—all of which are sugar-sweetened.

Paradoxically, a new HHFKA requirement that kids be served fruit at breakfast only adds to the sugar overload. Although most districts do serve fresh fruit at least a few days a week, they can also meet the requirement with canned fruit in light sugar syrup, as well as with dried fruit, some of which is allowed to contain added sugar. And up to half the time, districts are allowed to substitute 100 percent fruit juice in place of actual fruit, an option which most districts eagerly embrace: juice requires no prep, is shelf-stable, and is universally popular with kids. But health experts say that juice and fruit aren't interchangeable, due to juice's relative lack of fiber and high concentration of free sugar.*

When all of these factors come into play, it's entirely possible for the majority of calories in a child's school breakfast to come from sugar. An elementary school student in Broward County, Florida, for example, can currently select a breakfast of sweetened yogurt and "chocolate chip crisps" (a single entrée); sweetened, dried cranberries; and chocolate milk. That adds up to a whopping 55 grams, or *almost 14 teaspoons*, of added sugars—five more teaspoons than a 12-ounce can of Coke and far more than kids' recommended daily limit of 4 to 6 teaspoons. A child in Stamford, Connecticut, can choose a Pillsbury Cherry Frudel strudel bar, fruit juice, and chocolate milk for 34 grams, or 8.5 teaspoons, of added and free sugars. And kids can easily eat these sugar-bomb breakfasts several times a week, throughout the school year.

## Cafeteria "Copycats"

Whether at breakfast or lunch, the frequency with which kids are offered junk-food-branded items in the cafeteria, from Pop-Tarts to Domino's Smart Slice, is also troubling.

You might have thought the HHFKA would be the death knell for these kinds of products, but the processed-food industry was never going

---

* "Added sugar" is added to a product by the manufacturer. "Free sugar," the term preferred by the World Health Organization, includes both added sugar and the naturally occurring sugar found in syrups, honey, fruit juice, and fruit juice concentrates.

to cede its foothold in schools so easily—and not just because it wanted to preserve that revenue stream. Of equal importance is the fact that school children are an impressionable and entirely captive audience: Get your brand names in front of them early and often, the industry's thinking goes, and you have a purchaser for life.

So even before the HHFKA's regulations went into effect, manufacturers were already hard at work to create so-called "copycat" or "lookalike" foods and beverages. These products, like Froot Loops for Schools or Cheetos Flamin' Hot Fantastix, use the same trademarks and virtually the same packaging as their unhealthy counterparts—right down to appearances by Toucan Sam and Chester the Cheetah—but have been reformulated to meet HHFKA nutrition standards.

So what's the problem with copycat products, given that they do have an improved nutritional profile? For one thing, copycats taste almost exactly like their less-healthy versions, thanks to the wizardry of modern food science, so these products only reinforce kids' love of hyper-palatable, highly processed food. They also make healthier food an even harder sell: How many kids will buy an apple sold next to a rack of Doritos?

There's also the troubling issue of stigma. While some copycat foods are offered as part of the federally funded school meal, most are sold to kids through the cafeteria's à la carte line. By making this "cooler," more attractive food available only to kids with cash, socioeconomic divisions among students quickly become apparent—so much so that many economically disadvantaged kids (especially teens) would rather go hungry than be seen eating the regular school meal.

Most problematic of all: students have no clue that copycat food is formulated differently than the versions they see in convenience stores or at fast food chains. So each time they see these products in their schools, they receive a powerful, implicit message that this kind of branded fast food and junk food should be a normal part of their daily or weekly diet.

## "Letter of the Law" Meals

The food industry's fingerprints are all over the federal school meal program in other ways, too—including on the nutrition standards that shape the daily diets of millions of kids.

For example, when the new standards were being drafted in 2011, the USDA tried to follow an Institute of Medicine recommendation that school meals scale back on white potatoes, which are eaten far too frequently by American kids relative to other vegetables. But the nation's potato growers and frozen French-fry manufacturers would have none of it. Their aggressive lobbying campaign, along with an outcry from congressional representatives in potato-growing states, crushed the proposal.

The nation's cranberry growers were similarly upset that their dried fruit wouldn't make the cut due to its high sugar content. So now there's a carve-out in the rules allowing sweetened dried fruit when the sugar is required for "processing and/or palatability purposes." Whatever the health benefits of cranberries, though, they're surely overridden by the fact that a single, school-food sized packet of Craisins contains a child's entire daily quota for added sugars—a full 6 teaspoons.

But there's perhaps no more jarring example of the industry putting profits over kids' health than the USDA's attempt to close a loophole that had allowed schools to count the 2 tablespoons of tomato paste in a slice of pizza as a full serving of vegetables. An industry-led front group called the Coalition for Sustainable School Meal Programs vigorously lobbied to defeat the proposal, and it will surprise no one to learn that two of the front group's largest funders, ConAgra and Schwan, are major suppliers of school-food frozen pizza. Minnesota Senator Amy Klobuchar led the fight to preserve the loophole (can you guess in which state Schwan is based?), and she successfully persuaded her fellow Democrats to drop the issue. As comedian Jon Stewart summed up that particularly naked display of food industry lobbying power: "It's not democracy, it's DiGiorno."

Then there's the food industry's cozy relationship with the School Nutrition Association (SNA), a 58,000-member trade group for school food professionals. Fully half of the organization's $10 million annual operating budget reportedly comes from major industry "patrons" like PepsiCo, General Mills, ConAgra, Kellogg's, and Kraft Heinz. In exchange for their significant financial support, these industry titans and their products enjoy prime visibility at the association's huge annual trade show, attended by thousands of school nutrition directors on the hunt for new menu items.

I've never been able to see one of these trade shows in person, but here's how *Mother Jones* described the scene in 2014, two years after the HHFKA nutrition standards went into effect:

> The Pillsbury Doughboy was on hand for photo ops, as was Chester the Cheetah (the Cheetos mascot). Attendees...flocked toward...every kind of kid food one could imagine: tater tots, PB&Js with crusts pre-removed, toaster waffles with built-in syrup, and endless variations on the theme of breaded poultry: chicken tenders, chicken bites, chicken rings, chicken patties, and, of course, chicken nuggets.

If the crowds at SNA trade shows are any guide, most districts have no problem serving this kind of "letter of the law" food: products meeting HFFKA nutrition requirements while pandering to kids' worst eating habits. As Dan Ellnor, the head of nutrition services for Jefferson County Public Schools, Kentucky's largest district, told me, "I don't see copycat as a bad thing—serving healthier versions of kids' favorite foods. We're just catering to our customers and the culture that we live in."

When I pointed out that school food could help teach kids what healthy food is supposed to look like, Ellnor invoked the first federal school food law, the Richard B. Russell National School Lunch Act of 1946. That law's preamble is framed on his office wall, Ellnor told me, and in reading the statutory language over the phone, he pointed out that the words "nutrition education" don't appear. "When the Healthy, Hunger-Free Kids Act came around, I think they saw that as an opportunity to expand into education around food," Ellnor said. "And I think that's a very deeply needed thing. But you just went beyond what the original intent of the law was. If you want to do that, fund it. And that's kind of where we've run into the problem."

## A Missed Opportunity

Ellnor is correct that the 1946 law doesn't expressly mention school meals' potential as an educational tool, but the idea was clearly on the minds of some congressmen at the time.* A House Agriculture Committee report that same year noted that the "educational features of a properly chosen diet served at school should not be under-emphasized. Not only is the child taught what a good diet consists of, but his parents and family likewise are indirectly instructed."

In fact, this idea of "cafeteria as classroom" actually dates back to the late 1800s and early 1900s, when the very first school meals were dished up in this country. These early feeding programs sprang up independently in various cities after new compulsory school attendance laws resulted in a lot of impoverished kids showing up at school too hungry to learn. And even students with a few pennies in their pockets weren't necessarily better off. Those who weren't able to pack a lunch or go home midday often turned to pushcarts, local stores, and even enterprising school janitors for less-than-healthy meals.

So women's groups and other charities stepped in, with the primary goal of filling the bellies of hungry school kids. But it was also understood that school meals would implicitly teach *all* children, not just those who were malnourished, about healthy food because, in the USDA's words in 1916, kids encountered them "during the hours set apart for education" when their minds were "in a receptive condition." As a result, these lessons in nutrition were being communicated "silently, to be sure, but effectively." The New York City Department of Education similarly noted in 1923 that even more important than school meals' nutritional value was their role in "teaching children what to eat."

And just as today's school meals could (ideally) serve as a counterweight to all the junk food kids are exposed to off campus, early school feeding programs had the same goal. A program in Cleveland, for example, was described as a way of keeping kids from the "dangers of food sold by corner groceries, push carts, and street vendors." And here's the USDA again, in 1916: "Every time a child buys food…on the streets he gets an inferior product and a harmful idea and a low standard of food quality and care; in the school he gets a wholesome product and, if properly planned, a helpful idea about food and its care."

---

* For the record, the 1946 law's "Declaration of Policy" envisions school meals as a means of: ensuring national security, "safeguarding the health and well-being of the Nation's children," and encouraging the consumption of domestic commodities.

Now imagine taking a group of early-twentieth-century school food providers on a tour of one of today's massive School Nutrition Association trade shows. What would these earnest social reformers think as they're greeted by Chester the Cheetah, then led past 850 booths, the majority of which are offering modern-day "pushcart" food—everything from tater tots to taquitos? We'd reassure our visitors that these products do meet school meal nutrition standards, but we'd also have to admit that no one lets kids in on that secret. Or, as one school nutrition director enthused in a promotional video for Domino's Smart Slice: "They don't even realize it's good for them."

And yet, remarkably, if we introduced our time-traveling tour group to many of today's school nutrition directors, they might find they're kindred spirits. On that same online forum for school nutrition directors, I recently threw out a question: *If you could change anything at all about today's school meal program, what would your three wishes be?* Here are some of the wishes that came flooding in:

+ "My dream is to have an integrated program where lunch isn't just a break from school, it's an integral part of a student's education."
+ "Connect kids to their food through gardens and farms. Serve real food. Make lunch/snack a part of the school's curriculum."
+ "I really just want to see more real food! I realize kids love items like Crispitos and chicken nuggets but I'd love to see made-from-scratch things...on menus."
+ "I'd love to give my kids more time to eat, to provide them with higher quality food, and to make sure they understand that your body needs certain nutrients to function properly and they can't all be found in a blue raspberry [frozen juice dessert]."

So what explains the huge gap between many school food professionals' dreams of educating kids about nutrition and their heat'n' eat reality?

## Money, Money, Money

School meal programs in this country are forced to operate like independent businesses—if those business were saddled with some uniquely difficult challenges. Ellnor, the school nutrition director in

Kentucky, ruefully describes his job this way: "It's like operating a full-service restaurant, but you're turning more tables than any other restaurant has ever done. And you do it five days a week, with your hands tied behind your back. While wearing a snorkel, six feet under water." In addition to the high food costs and overhead of a restaurant, school meal programs have to contend with insufficient funding, reams of regulations (no food service operation is more heavily regulated), often-woefully inadequate kitchens, and a notoriously fickle clientele.

School nutrition departments are also required to be self-sustaining, meaning they have to rely primarily on federal reimbursement, along with smaller state contributions, to run their meal programs. In 2018, that federal reimbursement ranged from 45 cents per lunch for children who pay full price for their meals to $3.46 per lunch for children who qualify for free meals. Districts also get access to free agricultural commodities—foods like grains, cheese, and frozen produce. This commodity food makes up about 15 to 20 percent of all the food served in kids' lunches across the country.

From this funding, along with lunch fees from paying students and any revenue earned from à la carte snack sales, districts are supposed to cover *everything* associated with running a meal program: employee salaries and benefits, as well as overhead costs like utilities, site maintenance, pest control, and garbage collection. And some districts even charge school nutrition departments more than their fair share for those services, just to help balance their own books. When all is said and done, most districts have about a dollar and change left over for the food itself.

"It's crazy," says Chef Ann Cooper, a school-food reform pioneer known as the "Renegade Lunch Lady" and the current school nutrition director in Boulder, Colorado. "We don't ask the math department to pay for itself, or the transportation department," yet school meal programs are left to financially sink or swim on their own. "You could make a case that you don't need buses to educate kids," Cooper points out, "but as a nation, we believe that if the kids aren't in school, then you can't educate them, so we pay for buses. But if kids aren't well nourished, they also can't be educated."

Faced with this intense financial pressure, school nutrition departments are constantly walking on a tightrope and the only thing keeping them from falling off is ensuring that enough children are regularly eating school meals. "Participation" is their holy grail, which makes school nutrition directors extremely skittish about menu changes that might send kids running in the other direction. So when health-conscious parents march into their office and demand that pizza and burgers be served less often, they're unwittingly asking that nutrition director to take a real financial risk—one she may feel she simply can't afford to take.

Instead, chronic underfunding pushes many districts in the exact opposite direction, toward the most kid-friendly, letter-of-the-law menus they can come up with—nutrition education be damned. It also creates a golden opportunity for the processed food industry. There's a reason why so many K–12 foodservice suppliers expressly dangle the prospect of "increased participation" in marketing materials for their copycat products, like the Kellogg's flier promising that its Frosted Flakes and Pop-Tarts are "the brands and products kids love" or the Domino's Smart Slice website reassuring cash-strapped nutrition directors that "Your lunch line will stretch farther than our cheese."

These aren't empty promises, either; junk food brand names really do get more customers in the door. In Ellnor's Kentucky district (and in many others), a popular entrée is the "walking taco": a bag of Doritos that's been ripped open and filled with chili and cheese. Ellnor uses school food-compliant, reduced-fat Doritos and a mix of ground beef and turkey in his chili, but to kids, it looks like unhealthy carnival food. Yet when Ellnor tried swapping out the junk-food-branded chips for a whole grain-rich tortilla, he got far fewer takers. Similarly, when I was critical of my own Houston district's decision to enter into a multi-million dollar contract with Domino's for Smart Slice pizza, our school nutrition director, Betti Wiggins, told me quite frankly that the Domino's branding was essential to her bottom line. "I don't know how to defeat it. They [students] see a box with a name on it, that's where they're going."

### An Impossible Dream?

Let's say a school nutrition director *is* willing to risk it all by serving only scratch-cooked, super-healthy meals, like the vegetarian curries and quinoa salads that celebrity chef Jamie Oliver prepared for students a few years ago on his *Food Revolution* television show. Would it even be possible?

Some districts in the United States do manage to pull it off, but for many, the best intentions just aren't enough. Here's why:

### Not Enough Hands on Deck

While it doesn't take a lot of highly skilled workers to open a can or heat up frozen food, preparing fresh meals from scratch requires a larger and better trained kitchen staff. But in some parts of the country, prevailing salaries for food workers are so high that schools lack the funds to hire the necessary labor; in others, the salary caps dictated by school districts are so unrealistically low that it's tough to find qualified applicants.

School nutrition director Anneliese Tanner runs a top-notch meal program in Austin, but she's the first to admit her local labor market makes it possible. "I'm proud of the work I do," she says, "but it's not just the director. You need staff, and here in Austin we have a big population so we can fill our positions with people with culinary skills. In a rural area, that might not be the case." And, indeed, one of the school nutrition directors responding to my "three wishes" question wrote with regret, "We have massive staffing shortages more often than not. Sometimes the labor required for scratch foods is just not there."

### My Kingdom for a Cutting Board

Then there's the problem of inadequate school kitchens. Freshly prepared meals require cold storage, space for food prep, and all the necessary kitchen equipment for cooking. But when the Pew Charitable Trusts asked districts in 2014 what they needed to prepare healthier school meals, 88 percent said they lacked at least one piece of necessary equipment—including very basic stuff like knives, scales, and ovens. Many also said they just needed more physical space. As a result, the Pew report found, districts all over the country were being forced to use work-arounds that were "expensive, inefficient, and unsustainable."

Congress stopped allocating funding to help school kitchens stay up-to-date in the 1980s. Three decades later, it appropriated $100 million for this purpose as part of the 2009 federal stimulus package, and it has since allocated an additional $25 to $30 million every year. That sounds great, but the 2014 Pew report pegged districts' total school kitchen infrastructure needs at $5 *billion* nationwide. At the current rate of annual federal funding, it would take around 150 years to close the remaining gap.

A lack of labor and kitchen equipment also affects what districts can do with their free agricultural commodities. Many of these foods, like unprocessed meats or frozen fruit, are healthy in their whole state. But because districts often can't prepare these commodities in their own inadequate or understaffed kitchens, about 50 percent of this free food is sent to outside manufacturers who do the cooking for them—including industry giants like Kraft Heinz, Del Monte, Campbell's, and Hormel. But when you ask the processed food industry to do the cooking, the result, predictably, is highly processed food. Commodity chicken in the hands of Tyson becomes a breaded nugget or fried chicken sandwich, while commodity cheese, flour, and tomato paste wind up being served to kids in the form of a ConAgra frozen pizza.

### Risky Business

There are a few other, less obvious forces pushing schools away from scratch cooking. One is food safety. Kids are especially vulnerable to food-borne illnesses, and when a worker is handling, say, raw poultry, there's a real risk of cross-contamination if that worker isn't properly trained. But when you're just warming up frozen nuggets in a convection oven, that's not an issue.

Districts are also routinely audited to make sure they're complying with school meal nutrition standards. That's a good thing, of course, but because of inaccurate measuring or other human error, a scratch-cooked meal might fail an audit. Processed foods created for the K–12 market, on the other hand, are actually guaranteed by their manufacturers to pass muster—and if they don't, the manufacturer, not the district, will pay any fines.

Justin Gagnon is CEO of Choicelunch, a Northern California company that sells school meals to participating districts. But while Choicelunch prides itself on offering kids a wide variety of fresher, healthier options, the company incurs huge headaches by forgoing highly processed foods and their audit guarantee. "The process of going through an audit with a couple of [processed] entrees and products on the menu is vastly less complex than going through that same audit with a wide variety of scratch-prepared entrees," Gagnon says. "The complexity of an audit increases exponentially the more you scratch cook and the more variety you have on your menu."

## Barely Enough Time to Chew

Finally, there's the absurdly—some would say cruelly—short period of time in which many school children are required to eat their meals. When children have a mere twenty minutes to wait in line for a meal, find a seat, and squeeze in some socializing—the reality in many districts—it's no surprise that schools offer a lot of hand-held, highly processed foods that can be quickly scarfed down.

"This idea that we're trying to feed kids in twenty minutes—we're not trying to feed them, we're barely fueling them," Cooper laments.

## Fierce Competition for Dollars and Taste Buds

If these challenges weren't enough, cafeterias also have to compete with all the other foods and drinks sold to kids on campus through vending machines, PTA-run school stores, and on-campus fundraisers. This so-called "competitive food" is now supposed to comply with the HHFKA's healthier Smart Snacks standards, but for reasons we'll explore in the next chapter, on-campus junk food sales are still rampant in many districts. And when a school cafeteria is forced to compete with junk food, it understandably creates a "race to the bottom" mentality.

Here's a perfect example: On that same online forum for school nutrition directors, one commenter recommended creating a breakfast "donut bar" where children can dip school-food compliant donuts into a sugar glaze, then coat them with cinnamon sugar, powdered sugar, or sweetened cereals like Cocoa Puffs and Lucky Charms. Hardly an ideal way to feed kids, right? But here was her rationale: "This bar does well. Competes with my school stores, which is good."

Competitive food also includes the à la carte snacks and drinks sold by the cafeteria itself to augment the meal program's too-meager funding. These offerings can be healthy, like yogurts and grab 'n' go salads, but they typically lean heavily on copycat items like branded ice cream and chips. It's easy to see why nutrition directors feel they have to resort to these sales, but if snacks drain customers from the main meal line and/or require labor to stock and sell them, the financial gain can be illusory. "They see it as the panacea," says Cooper, "but we often see people losing money on à la carte. However, just the amount of cash flow makes them feel like they have money."

Finally, another kind of competition that drains meal participation is the open campus. It's no coincidence that many schools, especially those in lower-income neighborhoods, are ringed by fast food outlets that can cater to kids before, during, and after school—while using such a heavy hand with salt, sugar, and fat that school cafeteria food seems bland and boring by comparison.

## If You Build It, Will They Come?

Even if a school nutrition director could overcome every single one of these crazy hurdles to create scratch-cooked, Jamie Oliver–style meals, there's still one last challenge: getting kids to actually eat them.

Here are some observations from the school nutrition directors answering my "three wishes" question:

+ "So many of my K–3 kids don't know what a fresh pineapple is, let alone tastes like. I had a kindergartener bite a banana without peeling it."
+ "They are so used to fast food items, it's hard to get them to try new things."
+ "In my K–3 level, even pizza that doesn't look that appealing beats out everything else."
+ "Given a choice between a beautifully prepared chicken breast and a reheated nugget, most kids are taking the nugget."

In other words, if kids are coming from homes where healthy food isn't the norm, it's asking an awful lot of them to make that leap in the cafeteria. And while classroom nutrition education could help bridge that gap, most American school kids receive, on average, a meager three to five hours of nutrition education a year.

As a result, even a progressive district like Cooper's can't completely abandon carnival food. While her menus do feature more adventurous, healthy dishes like Korean bibimbap or Japanese tofu ramen, about a third of her menu still consists of kid-food favorites like pizza, nachos, and hot dogs. (That said, Cooper's hot dogs are antibiotic- and nitrate-free, and her pizza and nachos are scratch-cooked from minimally processed ingredients.) Similarly, Tanner's program in Austin suffered a significant 2 percent drop in participation among elementary students when she instituted what she calls "a very aggressive menu, with a big focus on scratch-cooking and global flavors." She's since scaled back on some of those changes, while still trying to expose kids to new foods through an ongoing cafeteria sampling program.

"It's a complex dance that we do," says Cooper. "There's a balance between pushing the envelope and educating kids, and actually getting them to eat. We have hungry kids, and the most at-risk kids are the ones least likely to eat some of that [more adventurous] food. You can't have kids in school for six or seven hours and not eating at all."

\* \* \*

In light of these formidable obstacles, it's no wonder so few kids are getting truly healthy school meals cooked mainly from scratch. And when you do see a particularly exemplary school meal program, it's worth doing a little digging. You'll often find that the district isn't pulling it off solely through federal funding, but instead is getting some kind of outside financial help, whether from a philanthropic organization, a contribution from the district's general fund, or both. It's great that these districts are able to secure that additional funding, but passing around the hat is hardly a sustainable or scalable system that can be applied nationwide.

And of course, the kids most in need of better school meals may be living in the communities least able to kick in or find the extra cash to pay for them. Even without the disparities that outside funding can create, studies have shown that predominantly African American and Hispanic schools are less likely to offer fresh fruit than mostly white schools, while low-income schools are less likely to regularly offer salads as compared to higher-income schools.

These are all harsh realities, but I certainly don't want to paint an overly bleak picture of what's going on in America's school cafeterias. As Cooper notes, "Twenty years ago, no one cared about school food at all, and now there are groups working nationwide trying to make change."

Among the organizations she cites are her own Chef Ann Foundation, which helps districts decrease their reliance on processed foods, and the National Farm-to-School Network, which helps districts source more locally grown food. Cooper's foundation has also partnered with the produce industry and Whole Foods to form Salad Bars to Schools, a nonprofit that so far has donated over $14 million to help over 5,400 schools get their own salad bar. And at last count, over seven thousand schools have a school garden.

Districts are also starting to exploit their considerable market power. The Urban School Food Alliance, for example, allows the nation's largest urban districts to collectively pressure the industry to produce healthier food for the K–12 market. Among its successes: After a years-long effort, antibiotic-free chicken is now available for the first time through the government's commodity food program. "I feel like we're in the beginning of a tipping point," says Austin's Tanner, "where procurement is driving some manufacturers, certainly the big ones, to make changes to their products."

Cooper gives much of the credit for these positive changes to Michelle Obama. Although Cooper's own involvement in school food reform predates the Obama administration by a decade, she says that during the six years of the First Lady's Let's Move! initiative, Obama "helped those of us wanting to make change move much faster and feel very supported." Even the industry-funded School Nutrition Association hasn't been immune to these shifts. "When I got into this in 1999," Cooper recalls, "I was the crazy nutcase outlier. And now I speak at the SNA. So maybe twenty years from now, it'll be that much better—I hope."

But despite these definite bright spots, the majority of school districts still face daunting obstacles preventing them from regularly offering the fresher, scratch-cooked meals most health-conscious parents would like to see. And on the other side of the sneeze guard, nothing in today's food culture supports kids' eager embrace of those meals. So asking a school nutrition director in one of these districts to replace the pepperoni pizza with a tofu stir-fry can be like asking a third-grade teacher to start teaching calculus to eight-year-olds—even while refusing to provide calculus textbooks or calculators, *and* while allowing students to fire the teacher if they don't enjoy the new math lessons.

Who in their right mind would take the risk?

# 6

# JUST ONE TREAT

*Last week I ran errands with my three-year-old. In ten minutes,
she was offered a lollipop at the bank, the dry cleaner,
the gift shop, and the wine store. It was 11:45 on a Tuesday.*

~ MOM OF TWO, BRIARCLIFF MANOR, NEW YORK

Because I advocate for food policies to improve kids' health, people sometimes assume I'm a crazy militant who never lets her kids near sugar. But I actually love sharing sweets with my kids. We eat dessert often, and our two teens have some very definite opinions about Houston's best cupcakes and ice cream. My personal weakness is candy—pretty much anything chocolate-covered from Trader Joe's will do—and when Girl Scout cookie season rolls around, my husband has been known to stockpile an entire year's worth of Thin Mints in the freezer.

So given my own friendly relationship with sugar, I never imagined that one day I'd be angrily pounding out an anti-treat manifesto—a ten-point document that would make a splash on social media and be downloaded by hundreds of equally fed-up parents around the country. And

I hit my breaking point over an event that wasn't even particularly dramatic. The day before I wrote the manifesto, my son's fourth-grade teacher gave him a juice pouch and a handful of peppermint candies. Hardly a big deal in the scheme of things, right?

But it's the "scheme of things" that's the problem. Because while the Oxford Dictionary defines a "treat" as "an event or item that is out of the ordinary and gives great pleasure," today's parents will tell you that the "out of the ordinary" qualifier just doesn't seem to exist anymore. Children are "treated" at every turn, and the resulting junk food glut not only undermines their diets, it also robs health-conscious parents of the chance to indulge their kids themselves. How can you offer homemade cookies after school when your child is already in sugar shock?

If you don't have kids or if it's been a long time since they were in grade school, this may sound like an exaggeration. So as an illustration, consider this typical day in the life of your hypothetical fourth grader, one that highlights all the instances in which adults—some well-meaning, others with ulterior motives—ply her with "just one treat."

### 8:20 a.m.: The PTA Fundraiser

As your child leaves the carpool line to enter her school, she has to walk past a PTA fundraising table selling donut holes, muffins, and cups of hot cocoa. She has a dollar in her backpack, so she buys two jelly donut holes to eat on her way to class.

[*Two Dunkin' Donuts jelly Munchkins = 8 grams of sugar.*]

Fundraisers like these are a common way for student groups and PTAs to raise money for everything from the band's trip to Disneyland to desperately needed teaching supplies. The goals themselves are always laudable; who doesn't want to provide kids with enriching experiences and the essentials they need to learn? But while school fundraisers can include car washes and wrapping paper sales, nothing makes a buck faster and easier than selling junk food to kids.

School campuses used to be so awash in unhealthy food sales that these fundraisers might have been banned under the Healthy,

Hunger-Free Kids Act, the same federal law that improved school meals. But when that law was under debate in 2010, conservative politicians, including Sarah Palin, hit on an effective talking point. They said the legislation would abolish the beloved American tradition of school bake sales, with Fox News warning viewers they'd have to "[s]ay good-bye to homemade brownies and Rice Krispies treats" as soon as President Obama signed it. The uproar was so intense that then–agriculture secretary Tom Vilsack actually felt the need to write a letter to Congress promising that his agency would "consider special exemptions for occasional school-sponsored fundraisers such as bake sales." But when all was said and done, the final version of the law contained a huge loophole: states are now allowed to set any number of "exempt" days when junk food can be freely sold on school campuses.

Twenty states have declined to take advantage of this loophole, but others have exploited it to the fullest. Tennessee, for example, allows forty junk-food fundraising days per year, while Georgia allows thirty fundraisers that can last up to three days each—half the school year. Oklahoma allows thirty fundraisers, each of which can last up to fourteen days. (And yes, your math is correct: that collectively adds up to twice as many days as there are in a school year.) Then there's Arizona, arguably the winner in this race to the bottom: it currently imposes no restrictions on junk-food fundraisers, and instead reportedly grants "waivers" to any school group that wants to hold one.

Even when a state has chosen to ban junk food fundraising, though, what goes on at individual schools can be very different. Texas was actually a decade ahead of the federal government in banning most junk food from being sold during the school day, but when those state rules were in effect, the scene on the ground was another story. In Houston, many high school PTAs continued to set up daily fundraising tables at lunch to sell pizza, donuts, and entrées from fast food chains. These "food courts" were so lucrative that many principals not only turned a blind eye, they weren't even deterred when our state issued fines for their violations. The money flowed in so fast from these junk food sales—literally hundreds of thousands of dollars a year, collectively—the fines were seen as just the cost of doing business.

In fact, even two years after the *federal* fundraising rules had gone into effect, I attended a prospective family night at a local Houston high school where the principal stood on stage and proudly rattled off his school's selling points. To my dismay, one of them was the fact that his students are able to buy fast food lunches three times a week as part of a PTA fundraiser. Texas's "exempt days" rule allows this kind of junk food fundraising only six times a *year*.

## 9:45 a.m.: The Classroom Candy Reward

It's now mid-morning and your child's teacher can feel a serious headache coming on. Maybe his students are crashing from this morning's donuts-and-cocoa high, or maybe it's the beautiful fall day beckoning from the classroom windows, but the kids are getting noisy and restless.

So he reaches into his desk for a bag of fun-sized candy bars and waves it slowly in front of the class. With Pavlovian predictability, his students immediately settle down and train their eyes on the bag. "OK," he says, "I'm going to put some of our math problems up on the board. For every correct answer, you get to pick out a candy."

*[One fun-sized Milky Way bar = 10 grams of sugar.]*

Every district participating in the federal school meal program must have a "wellness policy" on file, one that includes a general nutrition standard for all classroom food, including food used as rewards and served at birthday celebrations and holiday parties. If it chooses, a district can also use the policy to ban food rewards entirely.

Because these revised wellness policy rules only went into effect in the 2017–2018 school year, there's no current information on how many districts have chosen to ditch food rewards. Even if we had that data, though, such surveys rarely drill down into the classroom to see whether individual teachers are actually following the rules.

But I can say this: when I conducted my reader survey in 2018, classroom food rewards were still very much a thing. A lot of parents echoed comments like this one, from a mom in Fraser, Missouri: "The school uses food as rewards way too much—Popsicles for this, gumballs for that, chip parties for good behavior." Recent articles in education journals, as well as downloadable teacher reward charts, also indicate that the practice persists.

Teachers and schools also use junk food incentives in other ways, from candy-filled "treasure chests" where kids can redeem points earned for good behavior, to class-wide pizza or ice cream parties for achieving some goal, like reading the most books in their grade or collecting the most Box Tops.

### 10:45 a.m.: The Classroom Snack

It's time for the class's mid-morning snack, which is provided by parents a rotating basis. Today's snack was sent in by a dad who thought he was doing a pretty good job by choosing a baked product with a modest calorie count.

[*100-calorie pack Nabisco Chips Ahoy! Thin Crisps baked chocolate chip cookie snacks = 7 grams of sugar.*]

In overcrowded schools, the cafeteria is often too small to accommodate every student at a normal lunch hour. As a result, some grades might be made to eat "lunch" in the morning—as early as 10 a.m.—or later in the afternoon. To keep these kids from flagging before a late lunch or after an early one, elementary schools often ask parents to send in a snack for the entire class.

But whether it's due to a lack of nutrition education, confusing product labeling, or a lack of guidance from the teacher, these snacks are sometimes so nutritionally poor that they amount to just one more "treat." As one of the moms responding to my survey lamented, "They ask for a 'healthy' snack but don't enforce this. So people bring in Oreo Dippers, cheese puffs, and Kool-Aid." Another parent echoed that sentiment, noting that her child's classroom snack "was supposed to be 'healthy,' but at that point my idea of 'healthy' was very different from most of the other parents there."

### 2:15 p.m.: A Candy-Coated Science Lesson

After a late lunch and recess, the class files back into the classroom for a science lesson: making molecules out of toothpicks and gumdrops. When the lesson is over, the kids gleefully disassemble their creations and gobble up the candy.

[*Six gumdrops = 10 grams of sugar.*]

Using candy and other junk food to make lessons more interesting is a relatively common classroom practice, at least according to my 2018 reader survey and comments left on *The Lunch Tray*. I've been told about kindergarteners counting with Froot Loops or M&M's, older students learning to graph with Teddy Grahams or gummy bears, and marshmallows used to build structures in STEM classes. One reader recounted a classroom holiday craft that involved making Christmas trees out of ice cream cones, cake frosting, and small candies. And my own (least) favorite example: to teach my daughter's fifth grade class about the circulatory system, the science teacher used corn syrup for the plasma, cinnamon candies for the red blood cells, and mini marshmallows for the white blood cells.

In each of these cases, art supplies or objects like buttons or coins would have sufficed. But teachers know that sugar captivates kids. As one math teacher has advised online, "Just the novelty of candy being part of a lesson (not to mention eating it at the end of the lesson) is enough to hold the attention of most children."

### 3:00 p.m.: The Birthday Cupcake

Earlier today, a classmate's mom dropped off a box of cupcakes in honor of her child's tenth birthday. With fifteen minutes left in the school day, the teacher passes them out and leads the kids in singing "Happy Birthday."

[*One birthday cupcake = 31 grams of sugar.*]

What could be more generous than sharing a birthday treat with classmates? But in a classroom of twenty-five kids and a 180-day school year, literally every week can include a Cupcake Day. (Some kids have summer birthdays, of course, but at least in my own children's elementary school, a few would bring in treats in May to avoid missing out on the fun.) One of my survey respondents said her child's school even allows celebrations for *half*-birthdays, and parents sometimes also send in juice pouches or candy-filled goody bags along with the cupcakes.

### An Alternate Scenario: Standardized Testing Day

Instead of a normal school day, what if your child had been scheduled to take a standardized test? In that case, she might have been offered snacks and drinks by the school—likely without your knowledge or permission—in an attempt to boost her test scores.

Testing day snacks can include protein-rich foods like cheese sticks, but schools often opt for "energy-boosting" foods like juice pouches and sugary granola bars. Peppermint candies have also been popular ever since a study came out claiming mint boosts attention. A particularly creative teacher commented on *The Lunch Tray* that she hands out Pop Rocks candy to encourage kids to "rock" the test, pieces of gum to get them to "chews" the right answers, and peppermint candies for "encouragemint." One elementary school was actually caffeinating its kids with Mountain Dew soda on testing days until parents complained.

[*Three Starlight peppermint candies and a Capri Sun Strawberry-Kiwi juice drink = 27 grams of sugar.*]

### 4:15 p.m.: Soccer Practice

The school day is over and your child has a soccer game. Her teammates' parents take turns bringing the snack, and today it's sliced oranges and Gatorade for halftime "refueling," then Rice Krispies Treats after the game.

[*One 12-ounce Gatorade Thirst Quencher + one Kellogg's Rice Krispies Treat = 29 grams of sugar.*]

According to a recent study from the University of Minnesota School of Public Health, snacks and drinks like these are one reason why kids who participate in youth sports leagues typically eat *more* junk food than kids who don't. Sugar-sweetened sports drinks like Gatorade and Powerade are a big part of the problem. The American Academy of Pediatrics says most kids don't exercise long or hard enough to need any hydration other than water, and that sports drinks contain too much added sugar. Still, according to a 2015 survey, 40 percent of parents still believe Gatorade is a healthy beverage for children.

Some parents are concerned about unhealthy team snacks, but others are unapologetic. In a 2018 survey of a group of Little League parents in California, several respondents told researchers that junk food snacks are fine because they're "like a reward for what they've done today" and that "you know, win or lose, they look forward [to it]." Interestingly, this same survey found that a least some parents bringing junk food would clean up their act if requested to do so by the coach or "team mom." But when those authority figures don't seem to care about nutrition, it can have the opposite effect. As one of the moms responding to my 2018 reader survey said, "The coaches set the tone when they provide a team snack consisting of Gatorade and a large bag of Doritos—at 10:00 a.m. Playing sports has introduced my child to junk foods he never even knew about, and he plays sports to be healthy. I wish coaches cared more about the contradictory message."

Whatever the motivation for offering them, unhealthy snacks can undo much of the health benefit of playing team sports. If she sits on the bench during at least part of a game, the average eight-year-old burns 150 calories in an hour of high-intensity sports—even as she typically consumes between 300 and 500 calories from sports snacks and drinks.

### 4:15 p.m.: School Clubs or Aftercare

Instead of going to soccer, your child might stay at school for aftercare or to participate in a school club. In that case, she'll likely be offered what one of my readers cleverly calls "Kid Kibble"—individually packaged, highly processed, dry snacks like Goldfish (*lots and lots* of Goldfish, according to my readers), pretzels, crackers, cookies, and chips.

[*One package of Pepperidge Farm Goldfish crackers = 0 grams of sugar, 18 grams of low-fiber, refined carbohydrates.*]

Sometimes highly processed packaged snacks are offered because of tight budgets or a lack of access to the kitchen space and refrigeration needed for healthier foods. But it's also temptingly easy for any activity organizer, even those who could do better, to buy several boxes of Kid Kibble at a warehouse store, stick them in a storage closet, and have afternoon snack taken care of for the rest of the semester.

If this snack is federally subsidized—which is true for most public schools' aftercare programs, as well as programs for at-risk kids—it does have to meet certain nutritional standards.* But while those standards look good on paper, they can still be met with pairings like 100 percent apple juice and a bag of enriched white-flour pretzels.

## 4:15 p.m.: An Afternoon with Grandparents

Instead of participating in an activity after school, let's say your child spends one afternoon a week with her grandparents.

Every family is different, of course, but I was surprised by how many readers mentioned "grandparents" as a persistent source of junk food in their children's lives. One mom told me, "Every Thursday, there's a caloric explosion after school. Her grandparents either take her out for frozen yogurt or they go to the bakery." Another mom reported, "My parents used to give my son brownies whenever they babysat, despite my specific request that they not give him cake or cookies. And then they totally lied about it! I couldn't believe it!"

There's actually a fair amount of scientific literature documenting this phenomenon, along with the tensions it can create between parents and grandparents. One representative finding from a 2016 study: "Nearly all participants—parents and grandparents—described grandparents as more likely than parents to provide preschoolers with candy, soda, and fast food on a regular basis. . . . [G]randparents spoke of holding certain 'privileges' and having the right to 'spoil' grandchildren with 'treats' as part

---

* Specifically, snacks funded by the federal Afterschool Snack Program or the Child and Adult Care Food Program have to contain two items from four possible components: milk; meat (or a meat alternate, like eggs, cheese, or peanut butter); fruits and vegetables (which can include 100 percent fruit juice); and whole-grain or enriched (refined) grain foods.

of grandparenting. . . . [and] as introducing a sense of fun and creating a closer bond with the child."

Who can begrudge Grandma or Grandpa a little indulgence? But even if a treat is bestowed with love, that doesn't make it healthier.

[*One four-inch brownie = 33 grams of sugar.*]

## 4:15 p.m.: Running Errands with a Parent

Let's say you instead picked up your child right after school and took her on a round of errands before heading home. If so, she might score some free sugar at almost every stop.

According to a recent industry survey, almost half of all dry-cleaners now offer some kind of free food—*dry-cleaners?*—with 38 percent reporting they offer candy. Grocery stores often have a kids' "snack table" set up at the store's entrance, and while many offer healthy items like fresh or dried fruit, some offer sweet treats. Other grocery stores offer children a free cookie if they stop by the bakery. Even some pediatricians' offices offer candy to reduce the stress of a visit.

I could go on, but it's easier to just list some of the many other places my readers identified as regular sources of free sweets in their kids' daily lives:

+ children's haircut salons
+ dance classes
+ occupational therapy
+ speech therapy
+ banks
+ swim lessons
+ tennis lessons
+ art lessons
+ open gym/kids' play spaces
+ churches and synagogues
+ car washes
+ obstetrician's offices
+ the post office
+ printing and copy shops

+ pharmacies
+ liquor stores
+ stationery stores
+ auto mechanics
+ various business offices
+ public libraries

Offering free sweets is actually a smart, inexpensive way for businesses to build goodwill. On a per-piece basis, bulk candy typically costs just a fraction of a penny—a pittance compared to the upside for business owners. According to market research commissioned by Spangler, the maker of Dum-Dum lollipops, 63 percent of adults said receiving free candy made them feel "appreciated as a customer" and nine out of ten said they preferred candy to any other giveaway, like pens or magnets. Another study even found that diners leave higher tips when a restaurant bill is offered with a few candy mints.

Children, meanwhile, are like little elephants in remembering which places offer sweets. My own kids were always suspiciously eager to accompany me to our local postal store, thanks to an ever-present basket of candy on the counter. One of my Twitter followers said her children beg to go to a particular restaurant "even though they don't like a single thing on its menu" because it hands out treat bags to children. According to Spangler's research, 58 percent of kids remember the specific businesses where they were given a Dum-Dum lollipop, and 42 percent of parents will return to those businesses as a result.

*[Two Dum-Dum lollipops = 7 grams of sugar.]*

\* \* \*

Depending on which activities filled her day, your child could have consumed anywhere from around 75 to 100 grams of sugar—an astonishing *18 to 25 teaspoons*—just from treats. (As we've discussed, children's recommended daily quota for added sugars is 4 to 6 teaspoons.) And of course, sugar consumption is only one measure of a child's poor diet; even if some of those treats had been savory snacks like chips or white flour crackers, she wouldn't be much better off.

I did stack the deck a bit by cramming a lot of treat-giving occasions into a single day—but only a bit. A mom in Los Angeles told me that at a recent soccer game, the parent in charge of snacks gave each player a bottle of Gatorade, two packages of fruit gummies, a Rice Krispies Treat, and two snack packs of M&M candies. An Indiana mom says it's not uncommon at her child's crowded school for two kids to bring in birthday treats on the same day. And a mom in Houston sent me a photo of her son's bowling league snacks—nothing but candy and cookies—adding in her email, "Oh, and kids can choose a soda to wash it down with."

And remember my anti-treat manifesto? Here's what was going on during that week in 2012 when I decided to write it. My daughter was in middle school and taking a few required weeks of German. We knew the teacher was fond of giving students food rewards, but I'd assumed this meant small amounts of candy to which I could turn a blind eye. Instead, he was routinely passing out full-sized bags of gummy bears, each containing five servings and 66 grams of sugar, as well as ice cream cups, Popsicles, and cans of soda that he kept in a mini fridge behind his desk.

During the week in question, my daughter asked this teacher for permission to go to the water fountain. Instead, he nonchalantly turned to his mini fridge and handed her a can of Coke. (Her comment to me later that day: "I like Coke, but he's made me sick of it. I didn't even want it!") During that same week, my son's elementary school held a school-wide lottery, which my son happened to win. His prize? A jumbo Hershey's bar with eight adult servings and 88 grams of sugar. And because it also happened to be standardized testing week, his teacher gave each student a Capri Sun juice pouch and, yes, a handful of peppermint candies.

Those innocuous peppermints were the straw that broke this mother's back. Here's the manifesto I quickly pounded out the next morning, which I pasted onto a stock "parchment" background and posted on my blog:

**The Lunch Tray's Food-in-the-Classroom Manifesto**

Food in the classroom:

+ Overrides parental consent.
+ Infringes on parents' freedom to feed their own children as they see fit.

- Contributes to childhood obesity, which now adversely affects one-third of America's children.
- If used as a reward, runs counter to the recommendations of leading medical organizations and potentially sets children up for a lifelong struggle with eating.
- Overrides children's own hunger cues, and encourages them to eat simply because food is presented to them.
- Puts food-allergic children at risk, or else excludes them.
- Deprives parents of the ability to enjoy their own treats with their children, if they are already fed sugar at school.
- Is a lazy and unimaginative way to reward children, who would be as delighted to receive a myriad of non-food treats (if we even feel tangible rewards are needed for academic performance, another question entirely).
- Undercuts the school's own nutrition education, if the food in question is not nutritious—and it rarely is.
- Turns the school into an adversary, not an ally, for parents struggling to feed their children well.

## PLEASE STOP FEEDING OUR CHILDREN

My manifesto clearly resonated with parents. More than one hundred comments quickly flooded in, the majority along the lines of this one: "Thank you for this. I thought I was one of the few parents who felt this way." Even teachers chimed in to thank me, because it turns out that many of them dislike the whole the birthday-cupcake tradition. An unopened box of cupcakes can be a constant distraction for students, they told me, and a lot of teaching time is lost in passing them out, waiting for them to be eaten, and cleaning up afterward. In the end, *The Lunch Tray*'s Food-in-the-Classroom manifesto has been downloaded so many times that I finally got rid of the parchment background because it was eating up everyone's printer ink.

I realize, however, that my manifesto is unlikely to prompt change unless a teacher or school is already open to its tenets. Too often, if a parent objects to a classroom candy reward, a pediatrician's lollipop, or a junky soccer snack, he's made to feel ridiculous for complaining about it.

Lacking a parent's-eye-view of a child's entire diet, outsiders only see a mom or dad who seems irrationally freaked out by a relatively small amount of junk food, leading to the conclusion: "Geez, you must be a total Food Nazi. Why should I take you seriously?"

There's another reason, too, why parents' complaints about treats fall on deaf ears: If we did put limits on all these treats, a lot of adults would lose the benefits they get from handing them out. Teachers who rely on candy rewards would have to forgo a quick and dirty method of maintaining order in the classroom. Soccer parents would have to spend more time in the kitchen cutting up orange slices instead of tossing a box of "fruit" snacks into the car. The PTA would have to hold more labor-intensive, and possibly less profitable, fundraisers—and so on.

The fact that so few adults are willing to make these trade-offs for children's health is depressing enough. But when viewed against the already shockingly poor diet of today's kids, which we'll explore in the next chapter, our society's collective refusal to re-examine that "one little treat" becomes even harder to swallow.

# 7

# BIGGER THAN OBESITY

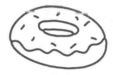

*He's filled with sugar at school and sports, and I worry about his weight.
Every year we go through a weight spike and then spend the
next six months getting it back under control.*

~ MOM OF ONE, AUSTIN, TEXAS

In a book about children and food, it may seem odd that it's taken me until Chapter 7 to talk about obesity.

With nearly one in three kids in America now overweight or obese, there's certainly no clearer measure of how toxic our children's food environment has become. In fact, based on current trends, Harvard researchers project that almost *60 percent* of today's children will be not just overweight but obese (that is, having a body mass index of 30 or higher) by the time they reach age thirty-five, compared to the current adult obesity rate of around 40 percent. And one expert has written that "even this bleak projection may underestimate the magnitude of the problem."

Kids' weight first started to skyrocket in the early 1980s, which means we've collectively lived through almost forty years of the phenomenon. Seeing overweight children—including, in many cases, our own— is now so common that, if anything, it's more unusual to encounter a group of kids who aren't overweight. "Excess weight has become the norm" in our society, agrees Dr. William Dietz, director of the Sumner M. Redstone Global Center for Prevention and Wellness at the George Washington University Milken School of Public Health. "You don't have to do anything but compare class pictures from twenty or thirty years ago to class pictures of second graders today," he says. "And [parents] may dismiss it by saying, 'Well, my child is a little overweight, but so is everybody else's. What's the big deal?'"

Diet is of course the most important factor affecting a child's weight. But we now know that genetics, socioeconomic status, activity level, and a child's overall environment play a role, too. There's even some evidence that weight may be affected by less obvious factors like antibiotic use, the endocrine-disrupting chemicals in some cleaning and personal-care products, and even viruses. The interplay between all these influences isn't fully understood, which is why scientists can't always explain why some kids gain excess weight while others don't—even when they live within the same family and eat the same diet.

And it's this last point that touches on why I've avoided discussing childhood obesity until now. Obesity is a public health crisis that deserves urgent attention, of course, but excess weight gain is arguably just one symptom of an even larger problem: that the *majority* of American children, not just those who are overweight, are eating a poor diet.

This sweeping statement may sound alarmist, especially in a country with such abundant food. Our ruthlessly efficient farms and feedlots produce 4,000 calories per person per day—far more than we actually need—and we spend a smaller percentage of our disposable income on food than the citizens of any other country. Our supermarkets boast an average of 50,000 products at any given time, with new ones constantly introduced to satisfy our every whim. But because so much of this bounty is highly processed and nutritionally poor, it creates a troubling paradox: children who are both overfed and undernourished.

# A Subpar Diet across the Board

In 2010, the American Heart Association rated the diets of American kids aged five to nineteen using its Healthy Diet Score, which has five measures: eating enough fruits and vegetables; eating fish twice a week; getting enough whole grains; not consuming excess sodium; and not consuming too many sugar-sweetened beverages. Admittedly, this is a high dietary bar even for adults, especially given Americans' general distaste for fish. But to achieve an "ideal" score, a child only needed to meet four out of five of those measures, while an "intermediate" score meant they were meeting two to three, and a "poor" score signified they were meeting just one or none.

The result? Less than one-half of one percent of American kids had an ideal diet and only 9 percent merited an intermediate score, which meant that 91 percent of American kids were eating a diet classified as affirmatively poor. Worse, the organization found that kids were eating even more poorly than adults, and that this troubling finding was consistent regardless of children's age, race, or gender.

It's important to note that even kids eating a poor diet are unlikely to suffer from severe nutrient deficiencies, thanks to widespread nutrient fortification in our food supply. It's also worth mentioning that this 2010 study was based on older dietary data (from 2005–2006) that predates recent nutritional improvements to school meals. But a more recent American Heart Association study of older kids (aged twelve to nineteen) using data from 2015–2016 is no less worrisome: zero percent of these older kids were eating an ideal diet, 10.6 percent had an intermediate diet score, and 89.4 percent had a diet classified as affirmatively poor.

Drilling down, we know that around 60 percent of the country's diet currently comes from highly processed foods, and that almost all American kids—regardless of their weight—are missing out in a big way on whole plant foods: vegetables, fruits, whole grains, legumes, and nuts. "It's not that children with obesity don't eat vegetables and all other children do," observes Dr. Jeffrey Schwimmer, a pediatric gastroenterologist and professor of clinical pediatrics at the UC San Diego School of Medicine. "The vast majority of children don't meet fruit and vegetable guidelines. It's fewer than 10 percent that do."

This dietary deficit is worrisome for two reasons. First, unlike highly processed products, whole or minimally-processed plant foods typically contain significant amounts of water and fiber. "It's that volume that regulates satiety," Dietz explains, meaning these foods fill us up and keep us from overeating.

Second, plant foods contain literally thousands of phytochemicals—the compounds that lend these foods their color, scent, and flavor—and some of these substances hold out real promise in preventing disease. Science is still trying to pin down exactly how phytochemicals work in the body, but it's clear that many of them offer antioxidant effects that help repair damage to DNA, improve immunity, and detoxify cancer-causing agents in the body. "These are all the things we don't yet know about that may have an impact on health," Dietz says. Yet the majority of our kids aren't reaping these potential disease-preventative benefits.

So if American children aren't getting enough of the good stuff like fruits and vegetables, what exactly are they eating? According to the latest federal data, the top six sources of calories among kids aged two to eighteen are:

+ burgers, sandwiches, and tacos;
+ desserts and sweet snacks;
+ sugar-sweetened beverages;
+ rice, pasta, and grain-based mixed dishes;
+ chips, crackers, and savory snacks; and
+ pizza.

Not exactly the diet anyone would choose to foster a child's health. And the really surprising thing is how early these poor eating habits take hold.

### Weaned on Fries

Between ages six and eight months, American babies are actually eating pretty well, according to federal data. As you might expect, their diet consists mainly of puréed fruits and vegetables, whole grain cereals, and breast milk or formula.

But when babies begin eating more table food, nutrition starts to takes a nosedive. At just nine to eleven months, American babies are already eating so many French fries that on a top-ten list of their most consumed vegetables, fries rank at number eight. Babies are also eating nearly two and a half teaspoons of added sugars a day, mostly from sugar-sweetened "juice drinks," cookies and brownies, yogurt, and higher-sugar cereals. (Experts say babies under age two shouldn't be consuming any added sugars.)

By age one, kids' diets are even more dicey. The second-highest source of vegetables for this age group is whole or mashed white potatoes. French fries now move up the top-ten list to the number seven spot, while potato chips make their first appearance at number ten. Close to 30 percent of one-year-olds are drinking sweetened beverages like juice drinks and soda, while almost 40 percent are eating brownies, cookies, crackers, and other salty snacks. Kids in this age group are now consuming more than five teaspoons of added sugar per day.

By now, you can probably guess the top two vegetables kids are eating at the twenty-three-month mark: French fries and potato chips. Meanwhile, 45 percent of toddlers are drinking sugar-sweetened beverages, and fully half of their fruit consumption is coming from some kind of juice. They're also now consuming over 9 teaspoons of added sugar a day—well over the recommended 4-to-6-tablespoon quota for kids over the age of two.

All of this is especially troubling because the foods eaten in the first two years of a child's life can affect their lifelong eating patterns. For example, babies who drink sugar-sweetened beverages on a daily basis, or who don't eat fruits and vegetables at least once daily, are more likely to be doing the same at age six. These findings hold true even after adjusting for factors like race, income, and whether the baby was breastfed.

Of course, the overly processed, sugar-heavy Standard American Diet (with its all-too-fitting "SAD" acronym) isn't doing adults any favors either. But there are some reasons why kids in particular are in the dietary crosshairs.

### A Sugar-Coated Crisis

All Americans have too much added sugar in their diets, but according to federal data, it's kids who are consuming the most.

For one thing, "kid food" grocery products tend to be sweet. As I mentioned earlier, when we look at all the new, kid-focused grocery items introduced since 2013, the largest category was savory snacks, but the next seven were candy, yogurt, juice, breakfast cereals, cereal bars, processed fruit products, and cookies. Even babies and toddlers are targeted by manufacturers with sugary foods, with half of the snack foods marketed for babies and 83 percent of snacks marketed for toddlers containing added sweeteners. Yogurt, a popular and seemingly healthy kids' breakfast and snack, can contain more sugar per serving than a brownie. And children's breakfast cereals are typically higher in sugar than adult cereals—maybe not coincidentally, since research shows kids tend to eat twice as much cereal when it's sweetened.

Then there's all the added sugar kids consume through sugar-sweetened drinks like soda, juice drinks, and sports drinks. Because they don't fill kids up, these beverages only add extra calories to their diets and are considered a major driver of obesity. Children's sugary drink consumption has dropped somewhat in recent years, which is good news. But despite an American Heart Association recommendation that kids drink no more than 8 ounces of sweetened beverages per week, 60 percent still drink at least one sweetened beverage on any given day, and about 30 percent drink two or more.

Even when parents want to rein in the sugar, the amount of hidden sweeteners in our food supply can make it challenging. In a 2018 study, more than three hundred parents were asked to guess how much sugar is in common kid foods such as orange juice, pizza, and ketchup. Almost 75 percent of them underestimated foods' sugar content, in some cases by a huge margin. The biggest errors, not surprisingly, were made with foods parents tend to think of as healthy, like yogurt and juice. And these miscalculations have real consequences: parents with the least accurate grasp of foods' sugar content tended to have children with the highest BMI scores. (This study took place in Germany, but there's no reason to think American parents are any better at playing "sugar detective.")

### The Juice Myth

As the German study indicated, juice is one of the foods that particularly confuses parents. Because it comes from fruit, many parents believe it's a healthy beverage for kids and a good alternative to soda. But according to most dietary experts, that health halo is undeserved. With relatively little fiber and around 10 teaspoons of naturally occurring sugar per serving, juice is actually closer to soda than it is to fruit.

In fact, the American Academy of Pediatrics advises parents to not give any juice to babies under the age of one, adding that older children should drink no more than 4 to 6 ounces daily. But according to federal data, even before babies are a year old, four of their top ten fruits are consumed in the form of some type of juice: apple juice, citrus juice, "baby juice" (typically grape or apple juice with added vitamin C, marketed by brands like Gerber), and "other fruit juice." By preschool, more than half of kids are drinking 10 ounces of juice a day, approximately twice the recommended limit.

Yet because of its "healthy" image, convenient packaging, and widespread popularity with children, it sometimes feels as if juice has become the default beverage for kids. Here are just a few of the exasperated comments I received from parents responding to my 2018 reader survey:

+ "My son doesn't drink juice at home but now gets juice daily for snack."
+ "When we tried to get healthy food offered at sports, the alternative was juice...not helpful!"
+ "Everyone is determined to give her juice.... Why?! What is the deal with juice?"

Even the federal government treats juice as healthy. It's permitted as a substitute for up to half the required fruits and vegetables in both the federal school breakfasts and lunch programs. It's also offered to families through WIC (the Special Supplemental Nutrition Program for Women, Infants, and Children), and kids participating in that program drink excessive amounts of juice compared to kids of the same income level who aren't WIC participants.

Oh, and when fast food chains and other restaurants get all that great publicity for improving their children's menus, they've almost always swapped out soda for...you guessed it: 100 percent fruit juice.

### Dining Out

Financially, if not nutritionally, restaurant children's menus are a good deal for families. A fast food kids' meal typically offers an entrée, side, drink, and dessert for around just three dollars, and even the more expensive kids' meals at full-service restaurants are still a relative bargain. Children's menus also offer parents another, less-talked-about benefit: the way their cheesy and fried offerings tend to keep kids content (or in the words of one candid restaurateur, "sedated") while the family dines out. Who among us hasn't bought a little peace and quiet in a restaurant with a free pack of crayons, a quesadilla, and a side of fries?

If eating out were restricted to special occasions, unhealthy kids' meals would be no big deal. But Americans now spend more on food eaten outside the home than on buying groceries, 25 percent of kids' calories come from sources outside the home (not including the food they eat at school), and just over a third of children now eat fast food on any given day. All of those statistics mean the food kids regularly encounter in restaurants can have a real impact on their health.

There have been improvements in recent years in the kids' side dishes offered by fast food chains (although only a minority of chains automatically bundle those healthier sides with the meal), and some fast casual restaurants, like Jason's Deli and Panera Bread, have made healthier children's meals a selling point. It's also true that eight major chains to date (Applebee's, McDonald's, Burger King, Panera Bread, Wendy's, IHOP, Jack in the Box, and Dairy Queen) have dropped sugary drinks like soda and lemonade as the default beverage in their kids' meals, meaning parents must now affirmatively request them for their child.

That said, the majority of major chains (74 percent) still have sugary drinks on their children's menus. And a 2016 study of the top two hundred restaurant chains found that the majority of children's entrées still exceeded a recommended 300-calorie limit, with one unidentified chain offering a child's entrée of two mini-cheeseburgers that provided a whopping 1,170 calories. The most popular children's side dish—French fries—typically contained triple the recommended 100-calorie limit for sides.

A key driver of those excess calories is portion size. The same 2016 study found that children's menu portions were often so large that the entrée alone exceeded the recommended maximum calories for the child's entire meal. And when presented with a too-large entrée, kids—just like adults—typically eat more food than they otherwise would. Researchers in 2003 found that when young children were offered an entrée twice the appropriate portion size for their age, they took larger bites and wound up eating 25 percent more of the entrée, but they didn't compensate for those extra calories by eating any less of the rest of the meal.

### Pizza. So Much Pizza.

I'm a pizza fanatic; I love it so much that when we lived in New York City, my husband and I would sometimes take a two-hour train ride to satisfy a craving for a particular pie in Connecticut. But when our kids were little, even I started to get seriously annoyed by the stacks of steaming pizza boxes that seemed to appear at every children's party or mealtime activity. I understood why everyone fell back on pizza for these gatherings, because I did it, too: it's hard to think of another hot meal that's as convenient, relatively inexpensive, and popular with kids. But the end result was that my children were sometimes eating pizza multiple times a week.

It turns out they weren't alone. According to a 2015 study coauthored by Dietz, the public health physician, one out of five American children and nearly a quarter of teens eat pizza on any given day. On those days, pizza accounts for between 22 and 26 percent of kids' total calories, and unfortunately children don't fully offset its bready, cheesy goodness by eating less at other meals. This net gain in pizza-driven calories (84 for kids and 230 for teens) can quickly add up to extra pounds—so much so that Dietz and others actually believe pizza is itself a significant contributor to the childhood obesity epidemic.

### Why a Healthy Weight Doesn't Always Equal Healthy

Fast food, pizza, and juice boxes don't make every kid obese, of course, but that's not necessarily cause for celebration. "One shouldn't have the mistaken notion that 'This child has a healthy weight, therefore they can eat whatever they want and have no risk of consequences because of it,'" warns Schwimmer, the pediatric gastroenterologist from UC San Diego School of Medicine. "There are those kids on the playground who eat nothing but junk food, and they seem very lean. But on the inside, it can be a totally different story."

One key factor is how children store fat in their bodies, which can vary widely. "Where fat is located is extremely important in terms of its impact," Schwimmer explains. "Fat that's farther away from the organs, particularly on the lower body and particularly closer to the skin's surface, tends to [cause less harm]. The closer fat is stored to the central organs, the more potentially problematic it is. And fat that's actually stored inside the organs—inside the liver, inside the pancreas, inside the heart cells— is even more toxic."

Excess fat in the liver is particularly worrisome because it's an independent risk factor for developing cardiometabolic diseases like type 2 diabetes. And when the amount of fat in the liver reaches at least five times the normal amount, the condition becomes nonalcoholic fatty liver disease (NAFLD)—with potentially severe consequences. According to Schwimmer, about 25 percent of children with NAFLD will develop hepatitis, and it's also the most common cause of cirrhosis, liver transplants, and liver-related deaths in young adults.

Thirty years ago, NAFLD didn't even have a name. But today it affects somewhere between five and eight million American children, according to Schwimmer, and Hispanic children are particularly at risk. And while no one knows for sure whether cases of pediatric NAFLD continue to be on the rise, the signs aren't good. In 2002, Schwimmer became the director of the Fatty Liver Clinic at Rady Children's Hospital in San Diego, the first clinic in the country dedicated to children with fatty liver. "When I started the clinic," he recalls, "it was just me seeing these children one half-day a week. And now we have four pediatric gastroenterologists and two nurse practitioners seeing children with various forms of fatty liver over eight to ten clinic sessions every week." In fact, according to one estimate, 25 million Americans will have the disease by 2025 and of those, five million will need a new liver. But that level of demand for donor organs can't possibly be met at our current rate of organ donation.

Environmental factors like air and water pollution appear to have some influence on the development and severity of NAFLD, but diet is clearly a major driver. "Added sugars in the diet increase the production of fat in the liver," says Schwimmer, "and low dietary quality is also associated with greater inflammation and more severe liver disease." So even when children aren't overweight, parents shouldn't blithely dismiss the poor quality of their diets. "We use weight as a focal point because it's easy to measure," says Schwimmer, "but it's really the health consequences that we care about. And parents need to understand that children can have some serious health problems without being obese."

## Junk Food Isn't Brain Food

Those are just some of the physical harms kids can suffer from poor nutrition—even when they don't gain excess weight. But an unhealthy diet can also affect kids' learning and mood:

### Classroom Crashes

Eating too much junk food doesn't guarantee a lackluster report card, of course, but there are a lot of studies strongly suggesting a correlation between diet and academic achievement. A 2008 study from Canada, for example, found a clear association between children's performance in school and their diet quality, while a 2009 review of over 160 studies also supported the common-sense notion that unhealthy eating may undermine cognition.

Sugary, refined-carb foods in particular—like, say, a school breakfast consisting of copycat Pop-Tarts, fruit juice, and chocolate milk—can negatively affect kids' learning in a number of ways:

First, these foods may actually stimulate hunger during the school day. Dr. David Ludwig is a professor of pediatrics at Harvard Medical School and the co-director of Boston Children's Hospital's New Balance Foundation Obesity Prevention Center. In 1999, Ludwig and his colleagues divided twelve obese teen boys into three groups: one group ate a high-glycemic (fast-digesting) meal of sweetened instant oats for both breakfast and lunch; the second group ate steel-cut (that is, less-processed) oats with a low-glycemic sweetener at both meals; a third group ate two slow-digesting meals each consisting of a vegetable omelet and fruit. In the afternoon, all the subjects were allowed to snack as much as they wanted. At the end of the day, the boys in the instant-oatmeal group wound up consuming a very significant 650 extra calories as compared to the omelet group. In other words: starting the school day with a toaster pastry or cereal and juice can lead to distracting hunger pangs mid-morning, and it may also set kids up to overeat later on.

A fast-digesting meal can detract from learning in another way, too: by causing blood sugar spikes that interfere with attention and concentration. As Ludwig describes it, "The brain needs a continuous, dependable supply of nutrients," but fast-digesting foods don't "stay in the bloodstream long enough to nourish the brain." As a result, he says, carb- and sugar-loaded kids will experience "surges and crashes that aren't going to be good for cognition."

These same foods also stimulate the area of the brain linked to cravings and addiction. In a fascinating 2013 study, Ludwig's team gave twelve obese men milkshakes, half of which contained uncooked corn starch, which is low-glycemic, and half of which contained corn syrup, which is high-glycemic. (The shakes were otherwise identical in terms of protein, calories, fat, and sweetness.) A few hours later, MRI brain scans of those who drank the high-glycemic shake showed increased activity in their nucleus accumbens—the same area of the brain associated with the abuse of alcohol, tobacco, and cocaine.

What does all this mean for kids at school? "If your addiction center and hunger centers are lighting up, that's going to be very distracting," Ludwig warns. "Kids' ability to exert executive function and focus on abstract concepts is obviously going to be limited." All of this raises the question: would at least some children currently taking medication for attention deficit disorder also benefit from a closer look at their daily diets?

### Mood and Food

Ludwig's findings explain why you have to peel your hyperactive kid off the ceiling after a candy-fueled Halloween party. But although the mechanisms are not yet clearly established, a consistently poor diet has also been correlated with more serious, longer-term harm to kids' mental health, including an increased risk of anxiety or depression.

And the mood-food correlation can work in the other direction as well. For example, we know that stress—certainly not unknown to today's kids—can increase cravings for junk food, which is why we all tend to reach for cookies over carrots after a difficult day. Not getting enough sleep can also ramp up sugar cravings. When researchers had a group of teenagers sleep just six hours a night—typical for many teens during the school week—they wound up eating more desserts and other sweets as compared to the days when they'd had nine hours of sleep.

## Childhood Obesity

All of these mental and physical consequences of poor diet can affect any child, regardless of his weight. But then there is, of course, the terrible and widespread problem of childhood obesity.

### Living Sicker and Dying Younger

I don't want to bludgeon you with statistics about obesity, many of which have been widely reported for years in the media. But here are just a few attesting to the epidemic's tragic health consequences for millions of American children:

+ Putting aside life-threatening diseases, the general quality of life of obese kids is often significantly impaired by conditions like joint pain, sleep apnea, asthma, and allergies.
+ One in three kids born today will develop type 2 diabetes in his lifetime, with all the complications that terrible disease can bring, including damage to the nerves, kidneys, feet, and eyes. For children of color, the risk of type 2 diabetes increases to one in *two*. And diabetes turns out to be a lot harder to treat in children than in adults, with kids more likely than adults to develop diabetes-related complications much earlier in life.
+ Obese children are more likely to develop other chronic diseases like heart disease, stroke, high blood pressure, gallbladder disease, and osteoarthritis. Obesity is also associated with a greater risk of developing Alzheimer's, as well as at least thirteen kinds of cancer. In fact, it's believed to be the second most important risk factor for cancer, after smoking.

In short, today's obese children are likely to live sicker and die younger than their parents' generation—a shocking outcome in one of the most advanced nations in the world.

## An Emotional Toll

Excess weight doesn't just harm kids physically; the associated stigma can also cause children real and sometimes severe emotional pain.

Overweight children are more likely to be bullied—and less likely to be offered help if they report the bullying. One recent study even found that being bullied as a teen correlates with obesity in later life, because kids may overeat to cope with the emotional pain of being stigmatized. Overweight children are also more likely to be viewed by their teachers as lazy, undisciplined, or less intelligent. And having to deal with this kind of weight prejudice on a daily basis takes a real toll: overweight and obese kids face an increased risk of depression, anxiety, and even suicide, and the constant emotional stress of dealing with weight stigma is itself a risk factor for developing chronic disease.

Helping children navigate this painful terrain can be difficult for parents. Eleanor,* an attorney in Chevy Chase, Maryland, was upset to hear her middle-school aged daughter recently berating herself over her excess weight. "She has a really good friend across the street who has always been very naturally thin, and my daughter's like, 'She's so skinny, and we all know I'm chubby,'" Eleanor recalls. "And it was frankly heartbreaking to hear her say it. I like to think she kind of compartmentalizes [her weight], but I realize that may be just wishful mother's thinking."

Deb, a registered dietician in the Los Angeles, says that even at age nine, her daughter is keenly conscious of her excess weight. "Oh, for sure [she's aware of it]," Deb said. "Absolutely aware. Acutely aware." And Deb, too, can't help noticing her daughter's physique and thinking about what it will mean for her future. "I can see her belly really protruding, and I have a visceral response," Deb says. "I worry about her health, but I also worry so much about ridicule and any sort of teasing and the fallout of not being in shape."

"Society is less kind to those who are overweight—all the research shows that," she adds. "If you're not tall, thin, and pretty, things just aren't as easy."

---

* Name changed at the interviewee's request.

According to many studies, a significant number of parents fail to recognize their child is overweight until he becomes obese, at which point it can be very hard to change course.

Sometimes this weight blindness reflects cultural biases—a bigger child is seen as "healthier," which is why parents are often less inclined to notice excess weight in boys—or it may be tied to a parent's own struggles with weight. Whatever the reason, this parental oversight makes it all the more critical that pediatricians raise the red flag early on, so families can make dietary and lifestyle changes before it's too late.

But doctors don't always speak up. Eleanor first learned her daughter was officially overweight when she saw her weight on the scale during a routine check up and realized she was no longer just at the high end of "normal" on the BMI chart. "I was like, 'Oh, crap. Now it's a health thing,'" Eleanor says. But surprisingly, the topic of her daughter's new weight classification was never directly raised by her daughter's pediatrician. "I kept thinking during the appointment, 'You're going to say something, right?'" Eleanor recalls. "But he didn't."

Eleanor's experience wasn't unusual, according to researchers. Doctors may avoid addressing child's weight for fear of causing offense, which is why the American Academy of Pediatrics recently issued guidance to help doctors navigate these potentially sensitive discussions. (Its overarching recommendation: focus solely on discussing behavior, like diet and exercise, without directly mentioning the child's weight, as the latter has been found to increase the risk of both eating disorders and obesity.) But other pediatricians may feel they simply lack the time in a routine appointment to address such a complex topic. As Dietz puts it, "The problem is that the pediatrician has fifteen minutes with a family, and they've got a big agenda to go through in terms of preventive care."

Failing to flag excess weight gain early enough can have serious consequences. "You run the risk," Dietz says, "that if you don't start counseling about [weight] until the kid's trajectory begins to increase, it may already be too late." That's because once a child becomes significantly overweight, he's statistically more likely to become an overweight or obese adult.

## How We Can Turn the Tide

Parents will always be primarily responsible for their children's diets, of course, and while far too many American parents lack basic access to affordable, healthy food, those with sufficient resources can strive to instill good eating habits in their kids. Parents can:

+ Teach children how to cook (or first teach themselves to how to cook, if needed), which is a critically important life skill in today's food environment,
+ Try to eat together as a family as often as possible,
+ Minimize kids' consumption of highly processed foods in favor of a mostly whole food diet,
+ Garden with kids—even if the "garden" is just pot of herbs in the kitchen—to help forge a deeper connection with food and its origins,
+ Limit children's screen time, not only because it's sedentary but because it invariably exposes them to more advertising for unhealthy foods and drinks, and
+ Teach children media literacy by expressly pointing out how food and beverage companies try to manipulate them through marketing.

But in offering these suggestions, I don't mean to lay the childhood obesity crisis at the feet of parents. If parents were solely to blame, it would necessarily mean there was a sudden, collective abdication of parental responsibility, across all ethnic groups and socioeconomic classes, mysteriously starting in the 1970s and 1980s. But of course, that makes no sense at all. As Dr. David Katz, founder and director of the Yale University Prevention Research Center, once wrote, "We have not a shred of evidence that the average, loving, busy parent of today is intrinsically less responsible than the average, loving, busy parent of yesterday. Yet that parent of today is far more likely to be obese and/or diabetic, and to have children who are obese and at risk for diabetes."

So what has changed over the last four decades? Nothing less than a "radical and toxic change in our food environment," according to a 2017 special report on obesity in the magazine of the Harvard T. H. Chan

School of Public Health. "The modern food era has spread out a smorgasbord of hyper-palatable, flavor-enhanced, additive-laced, convenient, and relatively affordable foods that are high in added sugar, unhealthy fats, and salt, and engineered to overcome our [internal] eating signals," the report went on to note. "Our bodies and brains are all but helpless in response."

And it's not just that we're surrounded 24/7 by cheap and delicious food. That food is also very aggressively marketed to us—and to our vulnerable kids. "The food industry brings in serious muscle to bully us into eating too much of all the wrong things," Katz writes. "Any conversation about personal responsibility or public policy that fails to acknowledge this reality is either disingenuous, or uninformed."

Scientists also now understand the biological mechanisms that make it so hard to lose excess weight, let alone it keep off. That knowledge is why many public health experts have concluded we should be focusing less on *intervention* and more on *prevention*: that is, making changes in our currently "obesogenic" society so the healthy choice becomes the easier choice. To that end, it's especially important to focus on children's food environments. "Preventing childhood obesity is the key to stopping this epidemic," the Harvard report noted. "By the time weight piles up in adulthood, it's usually too late."

But just because we clearly need sweeping measures to improve our larger food environment, individual moms and dads still have an important role to play. We parents are right there on the front lines of our kids' daily lives, from classrooms to cafeterias to baseball fields, which means we're uniquely positioned to advocate for change through face-to-face conversations with principals, coaches, and school nutrition directors. We also have real power as consumers: corporations do care about what parents think, and we can now communicate with them more easily, thanks to social media. And finally, parents willing to dedicate more time and energy can engage in bigger-picture food advocacy, by starting organizations in their own communities or supporting existing groups doing this important work.

So let's talk next about how parents can best advocate for their kids, advice that's based in part on my own experience as a very reluctant "accidental activist."

# 8

# PUSHING BACK

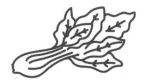

*If parents want to make it happen they need to team up—*
*strength is in numbers! We created a logo for our group and*
*ordered buttons to send a message that we meant business!*

~ A MOM COMMENTING ON *THE LUNCH TRAY*

The first time I was described as an "activist," it made my head spin.
To me, activism meant marches and demonstrations, a willingness
to get in people's faces, and having a very thick skin. I was grateful to
anyone willing to rabble-rouse like that for the causes I believed in, but it
was so *not* my style. I'd left my first job as a litigator precisely because
I disliked being combative, opting instead for an in-house legal job that
was more about collaboration than conflict.

It was writing about kids and food on *The Lunch Tray* that turned
me into an "accidental activist." The blog was just supposed to be a fun
writing outlet, and I enjoyed posting everything from children's cookbook
reviews to new ideas for lunchbox packing. But I did have some actual

opinions on weightier issues, like child-directed junk food advertising or subpar school meals, and when it came to those more serious posts, I instinctively drew on the skills I'd developed as a lawyer: doing my homework, looking at all sides of the issue, and then making my case as persuasively as I knew how. And maybe because I was trying to offer reasoned arguments instead of angry rants, those policy-related posts tended to be especially well received and shared on social media. Before long, I was having a small but gratifying influence on issues I cared about—yet always from behind the safety of my computer screen.

That changed in 2012. I had just launched my first Change.org petition, one focused on the use of "lean, finely textured beef" (LFTB), or what the media often called "pink slime," in school meals.* LFTB is made from slaughterhouse scraps, sometimes contaminated with cow feces, that are treated with ammonium hydroxide to kill the pathogens; my petition asked the U.S. Department of Agriculture (USDA) to stop providing schools with ground beef containing the product. I expected the petition to garner a few hundred signatures at most, but due to a barrage of national media coverage about LFTB generally, it unexpectedly caught fire: within just a matter of days, the petition had been signed by over a quarter of a million people. That's when the USDA changed its policy by offering school districts the option of ordering their commodity ground beef with or without LFTB.

Because of the intense interest in LFTB and the surprising success of my petition, I was suddenly doing things I never imagined I was capable of. I was a guest on Anderson Cooper's daytime talk show and interviewed on national news programs, and I engaged in weeks of heated public debate about LFTB on the Internet. I also became a target of beef industry supporters, many of whom flooded *The Lunch Tray* daily with angry comments—sometimes with unprintable misogynistic or anti-Semitic language and a few suggesting that the commenter knew where I lived.

It was a challenging experience, but one that demonstrated the real power of citizen activism. It inspired me to continue to advocate for

---

* The term "pink slime" wasn't coined by the media but instead by a USDA microbiologist who used that term to describe the product to his colleagues in an internal agency email. That email was later discovered by then–*New York Times* reporter Michael Moss, as part of his 2009 Pulitzer Prize–winning series on the beef industry.

various kid- and food-related causes and in the intervening years, I've worked to help improve the school food environment in my own Houston district and I've advocated nationally in support of federal school meal reform. With my friend and colleague, Nancy Fink Huehnergarth, I also launched a second Change.org petition in 2014. Working with food safety advocates and Connecticut congresswoman Rosa De Lauro, we sought to ban chicken processed in China—a country with a terrible food safety record—from school meals. Our petition garnered almost 330,000 signatures and, thanks to the efforts of concerned lawmakers like DeLauro and Maine congresswoman Chellie Pingree, Congress has since included language every year in the federal budget bill keeping this potentially dangerous food out of our children's cafeterias.

But the campaign I'm most proud of—the one that, more than any other, demonstrated to me the collective power of ordinary parents—took place in 2015. It began one fall morning at a local elementary school, where I'd been asked to join a panel discussion following a parent screening of *Fed Up*, a documentary about processed food. The film was already in progress when I arrived, and as I walked into the school's darkened auditorium, the event's organizer came over and whispered in my ear: another parent at the school had been unable to attend the screening, she said, and he'd asked her to make sure I received a folder of materials he'd left with her.

It was a puzzling exchange, but after sticking the folder in my bag, I forgot about it until I returned home later that morning. That's when I discovered that the parent in question was the president of the Houston-area McDonald's franchisee association, and that his packet contained a DVD of a film called *540 Meals: Choices Make the Difference* and a related "Teacher Discussion Guide." In a cover letter addressed to me, the franchisee explained that the film reflected McDonald's interest in promoting "nutrition education and awareness" and he was seeking my help in getting it shown in our district's middle and high schools.

"McDonald's" and "nutrition education" don't often appear in the same sentence, so I popped the DVD into my laptop, curious to learn what all this was about. When the film's credits rolled twenty minutes later, I was dumbfounded.

*540 Meals* appeared to be McDonald's decade-too-late rebuttal to the 2004 film *Super Size Me*, in which documentarian Morgan Spurlock ate McDonald's for thirty days and saw his health deteriorate. In McDonald's iteration of this same experiment, an Iowa science teacher named John Cisna ate nothing but McDonald's for six months and managed to lose 60 pounds.

Though he doesn't mention this in the film, Cisna says in an earlier self-published book, *My McDonald's Diet*, that he hatched the plan over dinner with a friend who happened to be a McDonald's franchisee. (The friend also provided the six months' worth of McDonald's meals free of charge.). And whether the company was alerted to Cisna's experiment by that franchisee, or whether it happened to see one of Cisna's YouTube videos about it, it's clear that the higher-ups at McDonald's quickly saw the PR possibilities in his story.

Before long, Cisna had quit his job as a high school teacher to become a paid McDonald's "brand ambassador," making the rounds on shows like *Today* and touring schools around the country to tell students about his experience. But there are only so many schools one man can visit each year and by using Cisna's amateur video footage of his experiment to create *540 Meals*, McDonald's clearly aimed to get his story in front of as many kids as possible.

The basic premise of *540 Meals* is that if a person carefully counts calories and caps his intake below his daily energy needs, he can eat anything he wants—even fast food. This "calorie-balancing" message has long been a favorite talking point of the processed- and fast-food industries because: (a) it puts the onus for weight gain entirely on consumers, ignoring these industries' relentless marketing of enticing but unhealthy products; (b) it falsely implies that, so long as a person exercises, she can eat without much restraint (we're never told, for example, that a person would have to run almost an hour to burn off the calories in a single soda); and (c) it conveniently underplays the whole matter of, you know, actual nutrition.

Yet *540 Meals* was even more troubling than the industry's usual calorie-balancing shtick. For one thing, the movie was intended for kids as young as eleven, and it was meant to be seen in *schools*, where students are entitled to unbiased facts rather than the self-serving messaging of a for-profit business. The film also featured a teacher, adding yet another layer powerful layer of implied credibility. Even so, I still might not have been that alarmed by *540 Meals* if it had offered kids an accurate discussion of calories, nutrition, and weight loss. Instead, it could fairly be characterized as a highly misleading McDonald's infomercial.

The central flaw of *540 Meals* was that Cisna never explained to kids that, because he started the experiment at a clinically obese 280 pounds, his daily caloric needs were so high that he could indeed lose weight on a steady diet of fast food. The same wouldn't be true of, say, a high school girl of normal weight, for whom a single meal of a Big Mac, fries, and a shake could constitute the majority of her day's calorie quota. And while it's true that Cisna told young viewers they would need "planning and mindful choices" to be able to eat regularly at McDonald's, he never offered the slightest hint about what that would entail, such as telling students they'd need a calorie calculator to figure out their own caloric needs based on their age, weight, and activity level.

Instead, in an era of widespread childhood obesity, the implicit takeaway of *540 Meals* was that kids could eat frequently and freely at McDonald's without consequence. Speaking to the camera, Cisna crowed: "Some of the skeptics said, 'Well, he only ate salads.' No. I had everything. I had Big Macs, I had the Habanero, I had Quarter Pounders with Cheese, I had ice cream cones, I had sundaes. And what's really amazing, that people find unbelievable, is probably 95 percent of every day, I had French fries. I love French fries and that was a great part of it."

The film was also rife with misleading, overtly pro-McDonald's statements, such as Cisna telling kids, "There's nothing wrong with fast food. There's nothing wrong with McDonald's." He also warned students that they should disregard any negative statements about McDonald's on the Internet, because everything on the Internet (including, ostensibly, science-based dietary advice) is inherently untrustworthy. To drive that point home, he even offered up a familiar quote about newspapers, a quote which he misattributed to Mark Twain and tweaked for the modern era: "A person who doesn't read the Internet is uninformed. The person who *does* read the Internet is misinformed."

It was this last, unbelievably self-serving admonition that pushed me over the edge. I searched online for the film as soon as I finished watching it, hoping to at least draw some comfort and validation from the scathing criticism I was sure I'd find. But the Internet was eerily quiet. The only mentions of 540 Meals were in a recent press release from a group of McDonald's franchisees in the Northeast and a short description of the film from a branding expert who'd recently seen it.

That's when it dawned on me that I was likely one of the first people in the country, outside of the McDonald's organization, to know about the company's alarming plan to get this film into schools. And if I acted fast enough, maybe I could stop this plan in its tracks.

Over the next few days, I did pretty much everything one mom sitting in her kitchen could do to draw attention to the issue. First, I wrote a lengthy blog post about 540 Meals, painstakingly dissecting the film and laying out every possible objection to it. My hope was that this post would serve as a useful guide for any reporter taking interest in the film, which is why I also sent the link to every media contact and outlet I could think of, as well as tweeting it to my followers. I also sent the post to two organizations I hoped would support my cause—Campaign for a Commercial-Free Childhood and Corporate Accountability International, both of which have long opposed McDonald's various in-school marketing efforts.

This outreach worked. Within twenty-four hours, the 540 Meals story had been picked up by a few smaller media sites, and by the end of the first week, pieces about Cisna and the film had appeared in major news outlets both in and outside the United States, including CBS News, Reuters, Business Insider, Gawker, and Mother Jones.

I was thrilled by this prominent, mostly negative coverage of 540 Meals, and I naively hoped it would embarrass McDonald's into retreat. Instead, the company seemed eager to double down, with a McDonald's spokesperson telling Reuters it continued to stand by the effort and Cisna telling CBS News he couldn't fathom why anyone would object to it.

That's when I decided the company needed to hear the voices of concerned parents, so I launched my third Change.org petition, this time asking McDonald's CEO to stop pushing 540 Meals into our children's schools. To help expand the petition's reach, both the Campaign for a Commercial-Free Childhood and Corporate Accountability International offered to share it with their respective mailing lists—support for which I was incredibly grateful.

Five days later, a particularly damning piece about 540 Meals and McDonald's other aggressive in-school marketing practices appeared on the front page of the *Washington Post*. Published under the headline, "How McDonald's Is Using Schools to Try to Change What Kids Eat," the story quoted me, linked to my initial blog post, and included a mention of the new petition. Because of that prominent coverage, I was later contacted by producers from both *Today* and *The Doctors* talk show, which allowed me to make my case on national television.

In both of those television appearances, I was pitted against a woman named Shaye Arluk, one of McDonald's many paid nutritionists. Arluk predictably defended the film and Cisna's school appearances, but I noticed that between the *Today* show segment and the *Doctors* taping, something significant had changed. While we were filming *The Doctors*, Arluk said on camera that *540 Meals* was "never meant to be ... nutrition education"—even though that's *exactly* how McDonald's had been pitching the film in its PR materials and to schools around the country.

That's the moment when I first suspected our petition had actually succeeded. And when I later looked at Cisna's Twitter feed, I became even more certain. Before our petition campaign started, Cisna had been tweeting every few days from speaking engagements at middle and high schools around the country. Soon after the petition launched, Cisna had abruptly stopped tweeting. When he resumed fifty days later, there were no further mentions of speaking engagements at schools, only appearances before groups of adults.

But until McDonald's publicly waved a white flag—which I knew it would never willingly do—I couldn't tell the 90,000 people who'd signed my petition that we'd actually won. Over the next few months, I contacted several reporters to encourage them to find out what had happened, but they either weren't interested in the story or they did some digging and came up short. And I knew I could hardly call McDonald's offices myself to ask, "Hey, I'm the person who started a petition against you. Can you tell me if we've won?"

Finally, nine months after our petition launched, the same *Washington Post* reporter who'd written the front page story wrote a follow-up piece entitled "McDonald's Quietly Ended Controversial Program That Was Making Parents and Teachers Uncomfortable." Somehow, he'd managed to get McDonald's to admit on the record that Cisna had indeed made his last school appearance right around the launch of our petition. Even better, the company told the *Post* that it had pulled the plug on the entire Cisna/*540 Meals* program, stating that "[n]either the documentary, nor any of the accompanying materials are being shared with or used at schools anymore."

In other words: VICTORY! And not just any victory, but one achieved by ordinary parents and other concerned individuals against one of the largest, most powerful corporations on the planet. Awesome, right?

## Flexing Muscle in the Marketplace

What the *540 Meals* campaign demonstrates is that when parents are a significant part of a company's customer base, as is the case with McDonald's, the company has every incentive to pay attention to our concerns. And with social media, it's never been easier to let corporations know what's on our minds. Just one viral tweet or Facebook post can make them sit up and take notice, and a viral petition sends an even more powerful message—particularly if, like the *540 Meals* petition, it also garners media coverage.

But even just communicating with a company via an old-fashioned letter or email can sometimes make a difference, says Dr. Marlene Schwartz, director of the Rudd Center for Food Policy & Obesity at the University of Connecticut. "In talking to food industry executives, I learned they really did pay attention when parents wrote letters," she says. "I was surprised at first, but I think people realize that when you take the time to write a letter, it's important to you. And particularly when they start getting multiple letters about the same issue, they really notice."

Corporations may be desperate to avoid bad PR, but the flip side is also true: they love looking like the good guy. And that positive reinforcement can set off a beneficial chain reaction. In the UK, for example, the grocery chain Waitrose voluntarily chose in 2018 to stop selling high-caffeine beverages like Red Bull to children under sixteen, garnering a lot of good press in the process. As Dan Parker, the former British ad executive, recounts, "And so the next supermarket thought, 'Hang on. I can get a good PR day here, too,' and then others quickly followed." Within just three months, Waitrose had been joined in its voluntary ban by seven other major grocery chains and one major drugstore chain. "And soon the laggards will be left with no choice, really," predicts Parker. "They'll start to look out of step."

For parents interested in waging any kind of social media campaign against a corporation or industry, here's my best advice: direct the campaign at just *one* decision maker or company, and keep your request as specific and narrowly focused as possible. A petition that says, "Processed food manufacturers—stop putting harmful chemicals in your products!" (that's based on a real example, by the way) will go precisely nowhere. No single company is going to feel the heat of that petition, and even if they wanted to comply with the petitioner's request, it's much too vague.

But a petition asking the CEO of Mars, Incorporated to stop using specific artificial food dyes in its M&M's chocolate candies very clearly puts the spotlight on *one* company and *one* practice. Just such a petition, co-launched in 2013 by mom Renee Shutters and the Center for Science in the Public Interest, garnered over 200,000 signatures. That viral response, along with associated media coverage, was at least partly responsible for the company's decision in early 2016 to remove *all* artificial food dyes from *all* of its candies sold in the United States.

## Improving Communities

In addition to getting our voices heard in the marketplace, parents can advocate to improve the food landscape for children in their own communities.

Lisa Helfman, for example, is a Houston mom and real estate attorney who in 2011 joined a Community Supported Agriculture (CSA) program. After noticing how the weekly influx of farm-fresh fruits and vegetables improved her young sons' eating habits, Helfman decided she wanted to recreate the CSA experience for kids and families who couldn't afford it.

So Helfman co-founded a nonprofit called Brighter Bites, which delivers free, unsold produce from nearby farmers and supermarkets to lower-income families. But instead of burdening parents with potentially unwanted and perishable food, Helfman was committed to delivering the produce in a way that might permanently change families' eating habits for the better.

To achieve that goal, Brighter Bites uses elementary schools in low-income areas as its distribution point, creating an entire educational program around the weekly afterschool produce pick-up. In a fun and festive atmosphere, parents and kids can watch cooking demos and eat samples of the finished product. Recipe cards for those same dishes are tucked into each bag of produce, which contain no less than eight to ten different varieties of fruit and vegetables each week—enough produce to feed a family of four. The program is also bolstered by state-approved classroom nutrition education for the kids, and parents are asked to help with the weekly produce sorting and bagging to get them further invested in the program.

Since its founding, a two-year, peer-reviewed study has found that Brighter Bites actually does improve families' eating habits, even when the free produce distributions come to an end. Thanks to that excellent report card, the program has attracted enough outside funding, both public and private, to expand to over sixty locations in four states—with no signs of slowing down. And what began as one mom's promising idea has led to the delivery of an astonishing 20 million pounds of free produce to date.

Lindsey Parsons is another example of a parent who decided to dive headfirst into food advocacy. When she realized the school food in her then-district of Montgomery County, Maryland, was sorely in need of improvement, Parsons co-founded Real Food for Kids—Montgomery (RFKM) in 2012. The organization began with just a few concerned parents gathered around a kitchen table, but it's now a school food reform powerhouse with over three thousand active members. As RFKM has grown, it's teamed up with other local groups to help elect school board members who care about healthier school meals, lobbied the state legislature to introduce bills to improve school food, and used its influence to help bring in a new school nutrition director who's more committed to scratch cooking and healthier à la carte.

Of course, not all parents are willing or able to throw themselves into full-scale advocacy projects like these. Sometimes all you want to do is get your kid's teacher to quit passing out Jolly Ranchers, or your fellow soccer parents to stick to fruit and water for half-time snack instead of Powerade and potato chips.

What's the best way to go about it?

## My Fourteen Rules for Effective Face-to-Face Advocacy

Odd as it may sound, I'm far more comfortable going head-to-head with powerful companies or industries than I ever was approaching the adults who plied my young kids with junk food. Many corporations so blatantly put profits over children's health, there's no ambiguity involved. But your child's teacher, day camp director, or soccer coach is usually acting out of motives that are entirely pure—or, at worst, only reflect some ignorance or laziness. What's the harm in using Tootsie Rolls in math lessons if they make learning more fun? My day camp doesn't have the staff to cut up fruit, but these vitamin C-fortified fruit snacks aren't so bad, are they? The ads say active kids need sports drinks to rehydrate, so what's the problem?

For that reason, I've often found face-to-face advocacy to be tricky, especially when it involves people like your child's principal, with whom you'll have to interact for years to come and whose help you may later need on some other issue. Instead of using a blunt instrument like an online petition, this kind of advocacy requires more finesse, thoughtfulness, and tact.

To help you navigate this potential mine field, I've created what I hope is a helpful set of fourteen rules for any aspiring parent advocate. This list draws not just on my decade of advocacy experience—including my many mistakes!—but also from interviews with several other moms who've successfully pushed for changes in their children's food environment.

### Rule #1: Don't Be a Fruitcake

Whenever someone in my children's elementary school plied them with unhealthy food, like the teacher who redeemed her good behavior "brownie points" with brownies, my first instinct was to just march into the classroom or principal's office without much forethought and share my concerns. But my success rate with this hot-headed, go-it-alone approach was pretty mixed. Those brownies were eventually swapped out for non-food treats, for example, but my repeated objections to birthday cupcakes and junk food holiday parties were politely dismissed.

Here's what I learned the hard way: just as my *540 Meals* petition turned one concerned mom's voice into the voices of 90,000 people, having three friends sitting next to you in the principal's office as you make your case is exponentially better than sitting there alone. Or, as a clever public schools advocate once put it:

1 parent = A fruitcake
2 parents = A fruitcake and friend
3 parents = Troublemakers
5 parents = "Let's have a meeting"
10 parents = "We'd better listen"
25 parents = "Our dear friends"
50 parents = A powerful organization

Indeed, every one of the successful parent advocates I interviewed for this chapter stressed the importance of "strength in numbers." Tish Ochoa, for example, is a Houston public school mom who was upset to learn that her district's school nutrition department was requiring her child's cafeteria to sell à la carte ice cream on a daily basis—even over the objections of the cafeteria manager. "Our district is over 80 percent Latino," Ochoa told me, "and we have a predisposition to diabetes. That's a concern for my community."

But Ochoa says parents should never advocate alone. "You have to be willing to talk to other parents, to say, 'This bothers me. Does this bother you? What are we going to do about it?'" In fact, Ochoa feels so strongly about "gathering your community," she says she would have dropped the ice cream issue entirely if it turned out she was the only parent who cared about it.

Not all parents would retreat so willingly, and that's OK, too—sometimes one strong voice is all it takes to get the job done. But flying solo is rarely preferable to having some wing-parents, and that's especially true when the issue you're trying to tackle is a complex one, like school food reform. As the late San Francisco school-food advocate Dana Woldow used to say, "Fixing school food is a team sport." Parsons, the school food reformer from Montgomery County, Maryland, agrees. "There are forces much deeper and bigger than you," she says. "You won't get it done with one meeting or one email, and you're not making change through one parent complaining."

Finding other parents to form your own successful advocacy team can be as simple as striking up casual conversations during school drop-off and pick-up, during soccer games, or wherever else you're hoping to improve your child's food environment. You might be surprised to find that many parents share your views but have been keeping quiet, assuming they had little choice but to accept the status quo. Some parents have told me they've even used online surveys to help gauge support for their particular issue, as well as to find potential allies.

Don't be afraid to look outside the parent box, too. You may discover, for example, that your school's nurse is an avid supporter of a junk food–free campus but just didn't have an avenue to express those concerns. Teachers, too, sometimes go along with customs like unhealthy holiday parties while silently wishing they didn't have to. And don't forget that your larger community has a stake in raising healthy future citizens. Depending on your issue, you may find support among medical or dental groups, in the business community, or with organizations in your area devoted to public health.

While bigger is always better, also keep in mind that you may need only a small core group of deeply committed parents, along with some others who may have less time but who can fill out your ranks. As Woldow advised, "If you can find six people who support your goal and are willing to help, ask each of them to identify just two other people who would... [be] willing to send out an email. That will give you almost twenty people who can be mustered in the event you need to make some noise."

### Rule #2: Don't Be a Hypocrite

This may go without saying, but if you expect other parents to clean up their junk food ways, you need to be willing to do the same. Yet I've learned from experience that sometimes this is easier said than done.

When my son was in third grade, he asked me to give a presentation to his class about Hanukkah. When I'd given the same presentation in the past for his older sister's classes, it had always revolved around food treats: latkes (fried potato pancakes) served with applesauce, and little gift bags containing a dreidel (a spinning top) and gelt (chocolate coins). Despite having written extensively about unhealthy food in children's classrooms, I actually found myself thinking in this instance, "Oh, come on, what's the harm in a little bit of chocolate and one potato pancake?"

Fortunately, I realized in time that it would be the height of hypocrisy for me to bring the food, so I just passed out the dreidels and my son's pleased classmates never knew what they were missing.

Moral of the story: You can hardly complain about other adults feeding your kid unhealthy food if you're part of the problem.

### Rule #3: Connect with Other Advocates

Before you plunge into any larger-scale advocacy, like school food reform, try to find out if anyone has gotten a head start on achieving your goal. You can ask around among other parents, talk to your PTA president or principal, call your district, look on the Internet for press accounts of any such efforts, or search the topic on Facebook to see if any groups have been formed there.

If you do discover that you're a latecomer to the cause, be sure to approach the existing group respectfully—and even with some gratitude for what they've already accomplished—before you start offering your own ideas. That humble approach will show you're a team player and instantly win you a group of allies. But taking the opposite approach can alienate the very people who could be your supporters. In the seven years I sat on Houston's school food parent advisory committee, nothing drove us "old-timers" crazier than when a new parent showed up at our meetings to complain about Houston's school food—but with no knowledge or appreciation of how much it had already improved, let alone a willingness to hear about how those changes were made or the obstacles still in our way.

### Rule #4: Be Informed

Effective advocates always take some time to bone up on their issue, knowing they'll need a solid grasp of what they're up against, along with useful facts and figures to bolster their position.

A great example is classroom candy rewards. At first glance, that doesn't seem like a topic requiring any research—we all know candy isn't good for kids—and it would be easy to just lodge a general complaint about candy rewards with your child's teacher or principal. But imagine how much more persuasive you'd be if you could calmly mention all the leading medical and pediatric groups condemning the practice, or if you could point to studies showing how these rewards can permanently harm children's relationship with food.

Parents concerned about unhealthy sports snacks can also get an assist from a little research. Sally Kuzemchak, a registered dietitian who writes at *Real Mom Nutrition,* coined the wonderful term "snacktivsm" to describe her own efforts to clean up the snacks in her sons' soccer league. "Knowing the facts is helpful if you get pushback," she told me. "The common refrain is 'But they're burning so many calories, a treat is fine!' yet research has been done showing kids don't burn nearly the number of calories playing sports that parents think they do." Kuzemchak also finds it useful to point out to coaches and fellow team parents that the American Academy of Pediatrics specifically states that most kids don't need sports drinks. Having all of this information at the ready shows "you're not just one lone uptight mom," she says. "There's research and policy guidance behind your concerns."

School food reform, in particular, is an area where a little learning goes a long way. You certainly don't need to become an expert on the complex National School Lunch Program; just having a general picture of how the program operates (which I offer in Chapter 5) will open your eyes to many of the challenges your district faces. If you're able to show your school nutrition director that you understand those challenges—or even just that you're willing to learn—you'll be miles ahead of that angry parent who marches into their office with big demands and zero clue.

Since kids' sugar overload is a common concern across many contexts, from day camps to classrooms, it's also generally useful to know the latest information about children and sugar. Many of the adults offering your child sugary foods and drinks may be unaware that there's now expert guidance on how much added sugar is too much for kids. They're also likely to be surprised—and hopefully a bit chastened—when you politely show them how easily their "one little treat" can exceed that daily limit.

### Rule #5: Know the Rules—Or Help Write Them

Educating yourself also means finding out whether there are any rules or regulations already in place addressing your concern. For example, does your child's sports league already have posted guidelines on its website requiring healthy half-time snacks, and those rules are just being ignored? If so, it'll be a lot easier to persuade fellow parents to swap out Oreos for orange slices if you have that policy at the ready.

Nowhere is this suggestion more important than in the school setting, whether your concerns relate to the food sold in the cafeteria, the food offered to kids in the classroom, school junk food fundraising, or the advertising of junk food on campus. That's because all of those issues are legally required to be addressed in what's called a "local school wellness policy," and every district participating in the federal school lunch or breakfast program has to have one.

Wellness policies have been around since 2004, but they were significantly strengthened under the Healthy, Hunger-Free Kids Act. As of the 2017-2018 school year, these policies need to articulate measurable goals for improving student wellness, along with reporting requirements to document the district's progress in meeting those goals. Every district and every individual school must appoint someone to oversee compliance with the policy, and wellness policies also have to include a nutritional standard for the food given away to kids in classrooms—including at holiday parties and birthday celebrations, as a classroom snack, or in the form of rewards.

This book's Appendix offers a wealth of information for parents interested in learning more about wellness policies, from their drafting to implementation, so I'll limit my discussion here. But one thing to keep in mind is that these policies are called "local" because they're meant to reflect the values of each individual district. So if there isn't a lot of community buy-in supporting health-promoting policies, your district's wellness policy may still be pretty lax. For example, a progressive district's policy might ban any type of classroom food reward, while a somewhat less progressive district might still allow food rewards as long they're Smart Snacks–compliant, which would include products like Rice Krispies Treats. And a community that doesn't care all that much about kids' health might expressly allow teachers to continue handing out candy, putting the onus on individual parents to opt their kid out in writing.

But precisely because these policies are meant to reflect local values, districts are required to seek the input of parents, students, physical education teachers, school health professionals, the school board, and the general public. This requirement creates a prime opportunity for parents interested in having some real influence over their district's wellness culture. Parents who would like to get involved can contact their district's wellness coordinator to learn more about the district's wellness council or committee, including how often it meets and how to join.

Although not required, individual schools can also have their own wellness policies, which are allowed to be stronger (though not weaker) than the district's. So interested parents can also work with their principal or PTA to set up a school-based wellness committee, which can then draft its own policy and help monitor compliance. In some districts, school-based wellness committees also send a liaison to the district's wellness committee meetings, which is a great way to foster communication between the two.

### Rule #6: Take Baby Steps

You may be bursting with big, bold plans for improving your child's food environment, and that's terrific. But the most effective advocates usually suggest taking on a series of smaller goals to slowly but surely change the status quo.

In the context of school food reform, Parsons advises parents: "Pick one thing you'd like to try and impact—but not something that turns the whole food operation upside down." In her organization's case, RFKM's first goal was getting artificial flavoring and coloring out of the à la carte foods sold in the district, not trying to revamp the entire meal program all at once. Another single, potentially achievable goal might be trying to install a certain number of new cafeteria salad bars per year, or increasing the number of school gardens in the district.

Sometimes, though, your discrete goal will get resistance from the other side because it creates financial risk, like asking your district to stop serving chocolate milk, which might decrease student participation in the meal program, or getting your local grocery store to stop stocking kid-eye-level candy in its checkout aisles, which might cut into sales. In that case, consider proposing a pilot program, like removing the chocolate milk at just one or two schools, or taking the candy out of just one checkout lane. Pilot programs are the parent advocate's best friend because they lessen the decision maker's financial risk while giving both of you a chance to study what works and what doesn't before you push for a full roll-out of the idea.

### Rule #7: Be Helpful

Sounding off about the junk food in your child's life can be very cathartic—trust me, I know—but if all you do is rant, don't expect anything to change. Instead, you have to be willing to put some sweat equity into fixing the problem. "Bring ideas and offer to help!" says Kuzemchak. "Too many times, parents gripe about something and expect someone else to fix it. Volunteer to get in there and get your hands dirty." In other words, if you're going to be the moving force behind, say, healthier Valentine's Day parties, you may also have to be the parent staying up until midnight putting heart-shaped melon pieces on little skewers.

Along these same lines, it's always good to pitch your proposed change as a helpful solution, not a burden. If your child's teacher often relies on candy to keep fidgety kids on task, for example, you could share research showing that "movement breaks" not only more effectively boost kids' attention and learning, they don't cost a thing and don't require a trip to the store. To improve sports snacks, Kuzemchak similarly advises, "Appeal to people's practical sides. Everyone welcomes something off their to-do list. Suggesting 'How about no snacks?' does that. So does asking for donations and volunteering to buy the snacks yourself—or suggesting people grab a bunch of bananas or bag of clementines and call it a day."

### Rule #8: Be (Really, Really) Persistent

One of Woldow's first pieces of advice to any aspiring parent advocate was, "You have to make the decision going in that, no matter what, you will never, ever, ever give up until you attain your goal." Woldow wasn't promoting stubbornness for its own sake, but for the powerful message it conveys to the other side. "You must make [them] realize that you are not going to give up and go away," she wrote. "Eventually they will realize that it is easier to just give you what you want."

When I asked Ochoa for her own best advice for advocates, she echoed Woldow's. "It's a situation where you can't give up, even when you keep hearing 'No,'" she says. "You keep pushing forward, with kindness." So, for example, in describing her own effort to get rid of the ice cream sales, she recalled, "Every week I said, 'OK, what's happening with this? What's going on with the ice cream?' You have to be nicely persistent, and if you really want something bad enough, and you ask and you ask and they realize you're not going away, there will be a resolution."

Or, as she added laughingly, "People get tired of people like me."

### Rule #9: Don't Be a Jerk

When your child is being offered unhealthy food against your wishes, it often stirs up strong, negative feelings. But experienced advocates urge parents to keep those emotions in check when pushing for change. "As much frustration and even anger that you feel," Kuzemchak says, "you have to approach it from a polite, calm position from the start, or you run the risk of having your concern dismissed outright. You don't want to be pegged as another angry, complaining parent."

Parsons agrees. In the context of school food, she says, "You don't want to come off as criticizing people because at the end of the day, you have to realize they're human beings with egos, and part of their ego is attached to the idea that they do their job well," she says. "So if you say, 'You're doing your job poorly,' they're not going to like you and they won't want to work with you. You have to walk a fine line of being collaborative and pleasant and making them look good."

### Rule #10: Don't Go over People's Heads

If you already have a good relationship with a principal, school board member, superintendent, or other high-level authority figure, it can be all too tempting to "go straight to the top" with your concerns. But successful parent advocates say it's always better to give the person closest to the issue a chance to work with you, only moving up the ladder if they refuse to budge.

When Ochoa was fighting her ice cream battle, she started with her principal, who turned out to be receptive to her position. "If I hadn't gotten any traction with the principal," she told me, "I would have gone up the chain further. But so many people get frustrated and want to jump to the top, and that can alienate your community."

And sometimes "the top" isn't even the best place to make your case. "My own efforts to bring change on the league level here in my community crashed and burned," Kuzemchak says of her efforts to clean up sports snacks. "My concerns were quickly dismissed as infringing on parents' rights. So I chose to go team by team. Each season I would approach the coach before the start of the season and ask him or her if they would be on board with just fruit and water for the season," she says. "Getting the coach on board is also crucial because parents will listen to the coach, while they won't always listen to a well-meaning team parent."

*Rule #11: Be Generous in Victory*

If you do succeed in achieving your goal, you'll likely want to spread the word, whether through word of mouth for smaller issues, or through a formal press release for the big stuff. Whatever the medium, be sure to share the credit widely—especially with "the other side." Parsons says that whenever her organization succeeded in getting any improvements made in her district's school meal program, "we put out a joint press release with Food and Nutrition Services to say, 'We both worked together to do this great thing.'"

Not only is sharing credit the classy thing to do, it can also lay the groundwork for future reform. As Woldow explained with her characteristic wit, "[i]t is vital to tell the public that [those on the other side] value student health and good nutrition for kids above all else (especially if you feel that they only gave you what you wanted grudgingly and maybe they don't really value student health) because once you have announced it to the world, what the hell are they going to do—say they DON'T value student health?" Burnishing the other side's public image has strategic value, Woldow said, because it "makes it so much easier when you go back to them in another month and ask for the next thing on your list. They need to understand that the decisions they make about your requests are going to be made very public, and that they can be the hero and support better food for kids, or it can go the other way and the public will hear about and react to that, too."

*Rule #12: Understand the Power (and Pitfalls) of Negative Press*

As Woldow's advice makes clear, both the prospect of good press and the threat of negative press can motivate a decision maker to do the right thing by kids—and sometimes, frankly, the latter is the most effective way to get the job done.

Parsons, for example, explained how her organization and twenty others formed a group called Healthy School Food Maryland for the express purpose of issuing annual school food "report cards" to every district in the state. Why? Because the prospect of a bad grade, which is likely to be reported in local media, creates a strong incentive for school nutrition departments to do better.

Even Ochoa, who generally prefers a softer approach in her advocacy (she told me she typically avoids being "forceful, or acting like an agitator") has used the threat of negative press to her advantage. When a meeting between concerned parents and Houston ISD representatives regarding the ice cream sales seemed to be going nowhere, Ochoa decided to start recording it on her phone—and she intentionally did so in full view of the district's representatives. "Honestly, I think we would still be selling the ice cream if I hadn't set my phone to record them," she told me. "Sometimes [in our district] it feels like only when there's the threat of media attention or negative press is action taken."

But if you do plan to share negative information with the press, carefully consider the bridges you might burn in the process. No one likes to see themselves portrayed badly in the media, and once you've implemented this strategy, there's no going back.

### Rule #13: Know When to Fold

The unfortunate corollary to "strength in numbers" is that if your larger parent community doesn't support, or even actively opposes, your goal, there's only so much you can do.

One of my *Lunch Tray* readers, for example, lived in a small, rural area where her child's school was awash in junk food. But her community wasn't remotely interested in change. Overweight children were considered by many adults as "healthy," she told me, while kids of normal weight were called "pencil-necked" or "beanpoles." She was even expressly told by a fellow PTA member, "We don't care about nutrition!"

Faced with that kind of opposition, it's probably time to abandon or at least scale back your goals. Instead of asking an indifferent or hostile principal to ban all junk food for birthday celebrations, for example, you might try asking if all children with a birthday in a given month could celebrate on the same day. And instead of pitching your proposal as a health issue, you might want to emphasize factors having nothing to do with nutrition, like the instructional time that's lost if, several times a month, a teacher has to pass out treats, wait for children to eat them and then clean up after them. In a hostile community, sometimes that kind of "reframing" can make all the difference.

### Rule #14: Take a Look at This Book's Appendix!

Really! My goal was to pack so much useful information into the Appendix that it alone would be worth this book's cover price. In addition to resources not mentioned here, it includes all the ones that were mentioned: that research on candy rewards and sports snacks, the latest advice on kids and sugar, information about wellness policies, and a trove of advice written by Woldow that's specifically tailored to parents interested in school food reform.

\* \* \*

In sharing these advocacy tips and resources, as well as the success stories of other parents, it's my sincere hope that you'll feel inspired, supported, and empowered. I firmly believe that we parents have an important role to play in improving our children's food environment—and that we can make a real difference.

But I also need to be straight with you. There are a lot of big picture problems directly and negatively affecting our children's health that are just too big for any one parent, or even any group of parents, to tackle. No matter how much we might want to see healthier, fresher food in every school cafeteria in America, the school lunch program isn't sufficiently funded, and most kitchens aren't properly outfitted, to make that a reality. No matter how much we might want to empower every parent to make the best food decisions for their children, that goal will be impossible so long as companies are allowed to blanket their product packaging with confusing and even intentionally misleading nutrition claims. And no matter how much we'd like to live in a world in which children are encouraged to make the healthiest choices, we're powerless against industries willing to spend $2 billion a year to market the least healthy foods and drinks to our kids, often using sophisticated digital techniques meant to fly under parents' radar.

There's only way we can address *those* problems and that's by taking our "strength in numbers" approach and putting it on steroids. That's called the ballot box. Let's see how we might use it to make our children's world a healthier, happier place.

# 9

# FOUR WISHES

*I feel like I'm fighting an uphill battle in this country
trying to instill healthy eating habits in my children.
At times it feels insurmountable.*

~ MOM OF TWO, NEWTOWN, CONNECTICUT

Today's food culture makes it so hard to raise healthy children that parents tend to forget: it doesn't have to be this way.

We could actually live in a world where kids could watch TV or play smartphone games without being targeted by ads for unhealthy foods and drinks. Children could pass through supermarket checkout aisles offering only healthy snacks, with candy still available elsewhere in the store. And students could eat in school cafeterias that don't feel as compelled to compete with junk food and fast food, instead offering more wholesome, homestyle meals. In other words, we could live in a world where we still have access to all the same delicious, if unhealthy, foods—

because really, who wants a future without pizza or ice cream?—but where the healthier choice would be the *easier* choice.

A list of proposals to make that world a reality could easily fill its own book. We could talk about sugar-sweetened drink taxes, which have already been adopted in a number of American cities, or shifts in federal Farm Bill spending that might make healthier food more available and affordable. We could explore the use of zoning laws to keep fast food chains away from schools, and the expansion of programs like the Minneapolis Healthy Corner Store initiative, in which corner stores in low-income neighborhoods committed to stocking and prominently displaying healthier foods, leading to an increase in customer demand. We could discuss building incentives into SNAP, the food stamp program, to give recipients more bang for their buck when they spend their benefits on fruits and vegetables. Or we could concentrate entirely on addressing the systemic poverty in our society that underlies so many health problems, including childhood obesity.

Those are all important and necessary conversations, but here I'd like to focus specifically on three major issues raised in this book: the marketing of junk food to kids, product marketing that confuses parents, and subpar school meals. I'd also like to explore ways of getting children invested in their own healthy eating—because unless kids have some skin in the game, any efforts to improve their food environment will be less effective.

Here, then, are four wishes for improving our children's lives and health, along with some ideas for making them a reality. These suggestions range from big-ticket proposals which would admittedly require a cultural sea change, to more modest course corrections we could make right now.

## Wish One: Ending Pester Power

Because the link between childhood obesity and kids' exposure to unhealthy food and drink marketing is now well established, addressing this marketing is imperative. Here's how we might do it:

### Ban It Outright

The most effective measure, of course, would be banning such child-directed marketing altogether, which is the recommendation of almost every leading public health expert and organization that has addressed the issue. The Harvard T. H. Chan School of Public Health says such a ban is "an urgently needed strategy," and that view is shared by organizations like the World Health Organization, UNICEF, and the World Medical Association. Apart from dietary concerns, the American Psychological Association and the American Academy of Pediatrics long ago issued their own statements condemning *all* advertising to younger children because it unfairly exploits them.

Banning such marketing may sound like a pipe dream, especially given the food and beverage industries' hold over our elected officials and their crushing defeat of previous such efforts. But I believe America's obesity-related healthcare costs will eventually become untenable, and that's when previously unthinkable solutions will start to seem a lot more reasonable.

This is exactly what happened recently in Chile. Alarmed by soaring healthcare costs that threatened its economy, Chile's government managed to overcome a decade of stiff industry opposition to finally ban children's junk food advertising—even including the use of brand mascots like Tony the Tiger and other cartoon characters on product packaging. And Chile isn't the only country to take this critical step. Peru, Mexico, Ecuador, South Korea, Taiwan, Turkey, the United Kingdom, and Denmark are among the countries that have in some way restricted or banned unhealthy food and beverage marketing to children, while other countries like Sweden and Norway, as well as the Canadian province of Quebec, have long banned all advertising to children, regardless of the product.

Here in America, the idea of curbing unhealthy food and beverage marketing to kids appears to have parental support, at least according to a 2015 survey conducted by the Rudd Center for Food Policy & Obesity at the University of Connecticut. Of the more than 3,600 parents surveyed by Rudd, 85 percent agreed that food companies should reduce the marketing of unhealthy food and beverages to children; 71 percent agreed that food companies don't act responsibly when they advertise to children; and 66 percent believed that food companies make it difficult for parents to raise healthy children.

Notably, these parents weren't just unhappy with the status quo; they were also comfortable with the idea of using regulation to change it. Seventy percent supported restricting unhealthy food and drink marketing to kids on TV and 66 percent supported the same restrictions in other media. Interestingly, parents who identified as politically conservative were actually more supportive of restricting unhealthy food and drink ads to kids under fourteen than were politically moderate parents (74 percent versus 69.5 percent), and were only slightly less supportive of the idea than liberal parents (76 percent).

Of course, not all American parents agree with this approach. Some moms and dads consider fending off kids' Pester Power a normal, if unpleasant, aspect of parenting. A common refrain from this camp is, "Kids don't drive themselves to McDonald's!" or "Children don't pay for the groceries!" But I don't see that view as at all inconsistent with a marketing ban. If you truly believe parents are the ultimate decision makers, doesn't it make perfect sense to ask companies to advertise *only* to you? There's just no legitimate reason why your kids should be dragged into the equation—especially now that we know this kind of marketing really does cause them harm.

### Use the Tax Code

Short of banning child-directed marketing for unhealthy foods and drinks, we could also use the tax code to help rein in these ads.
Corporations are currently allowed to deduct their advertising expenses—just like any other ordinary business expense—regardless of whether those ads happen to promote unhealthy foods and drinks to kids. According to Steven Gortmaker, a professor of the practice of health sociology and director of the Harvard Prevention Research Center on Nutrition and Physical Activity, eliminating the tax deduction just for companies' child-directed TV ads promoting unhealthy products could save $260 million in healthcare costs and prevent 129,100 cases of childhood obesity by 2025. Put another way, if we don't eliminate this deduction, we're essentially providing corporations with a government subsidy to engage in a practice known to harm children.

### Fight Fire with Fire

Even as we work to eliminate junk food ads for kids, we could also take a few pages from the industry's playbook to promote the healthy foods kids so sorely need.

We could, for example, fund a public health campaign using video games to shift kids eating behavior, just as the food industry uses such games to promote its own unhealthy products. When children played an advergame sponsored by the produce company Dole, for example, they later ate more fruits and vegetables and fewer salty snacks than kids who played an advergame featuring Pop-Tarts or Oreos. Another study found that children ate more healthfully after playing a video game in which they scored points every time a Pac-Man character ate healthy snacks.

We could also enlist beloved children's characters and popular celebrities and athletes, just like the industry does. That was the idea behind a deal brokered in 2013 by Michelle Obama's Partnership for a Healthier America, which allowed produce growers, suppliers, and retailers to use Sesame Street characters, free of charge, to promote fruit and vegetables to young children. Obama's organization is also behind "Team FNV," a slick marketing campaign aimed at older children and adults featuring an impressive roster of big names, including Stephen Curry, Jessica Alba, and Nick Jonas, to make "FNV"—fruits and vegetables—seem as hip and cool as the latest junk food.

Seventy-nine percent of parents in the Rudd survey liked the idea of requiring children's media companies to fund public service announcements promoting fruits and vegetables to kids, and that's where these proven marketing techniques could be put to use. But not everyone is on board with this plan. Josh Golin, executive director of the Campaign for a Commercial-Free Childhood, believes that "teaching kids to follow celebrities or characters or games or stickers"—even to encourage them to eat the healthy stuff—only further undermines their relationship with food. "We want to get them to eat for the right reasons," Golin says, which means listening to their own hunger cues and viewing "food as an experience we share with our families, not just another form of entertainment." He also points out that as long as the food industry continues its own use of celebrities and characters, we're only going to confuse kids even more. "How do we teach kids, 'It's OK to eat that banana because Elmo is on there, but not that sugary cereal with Dora on it'?" Golin warns.

Like Golin, I'd love to live in a world where all marketing to kids is off limits. But until that day comes, I'd be fine with using cartoon characters and other marketing hooks to get kids interested in just *one* particular category of healthy food: fresh or minimally processed fruits and vegetables. I make that important distinction because, as Michael Pollan advises in *Food Rules*, "If you're not hungry enough to eat an apple, then you're probably not hungry." In other words, it's easy to mindlessly overeat processed foods—even healthier ones, like whole-grain crackers—but it seems highly unlikely that a child will gorge herself on carrots and cantaloupe, no matter how much she loves Dora or Elmo.

If I'm wrong, I think most parents would happily take that "problem" over our current one.

## Wish Two: Help Kids Embrace Healthier Foods

As we work to improve our current, unhealthy food environment, we also need to arm children with knowledge and tools to successfully navigate the status quo.

This knowledge starts with improving children's basic food literacy. When chef and advocate Jamie Oliver visited a first-grade classroom in West Virginia in 2010, he discovered that while every student was well-acquainted with ketchup, not a single one could identify a fresh tomato. The same was true for other common fruits and vegetables, including cauliflower, beets, and eggplant. When Oliver spoke with Los Angeles high schoolers the following year, he found that many of them were just as confused. One high school senior thought honey was produced by bears, while another thought cheese came from pasta.

This degree of food illiteracy probably shouldn't surprise anyone, given that the majority of Americans' daily calories are now highly pro-cessed. But although we clearly need more classroom instruction to boost children's food IQ, we also have to recognize that abstract knowledge doesn't always translate into changed behavior. In a 2016 Pew survey, 97 percent of Americans recognized that healthy eating habits are very or somewhat important, but 58 percent admitted "most days I probably should be eating healthier."

So in addition to more effectively teaching kids the facts and figures of good nutrition, we should also fund initiatives like these:

## Bring Back Home Economics

Experts have long suspected that having cooking skills can make a real difference in people's eating habits, and a 2018 study backs them up. For ten years, the University of Minnesota's School of Public Health followed more than 1,100 young adults and found that those who reported having "very adequate" cooking skills at the start of the study were more likely a decade later to be preparing their own meals, including meals with vegetables, and they were less likely to regularly eat fast food. If they had families of their own, they were also more likely to eat family meals, thus setting their own kids on a healthier path.

With fewer parents preparing meals from scratch, though, kids can't always learn basic cooking skills through observation at home. And most schools no longer have classrooms outfitted for home economics, which is another way prior generations of Americans learned to fend for themselves in the kitchen. But there are ways around this problem. In 2014, the Charlie Cart Project held a successful Kickstarter campaign to help bring its compact, cleverly designed mobile kitchens to schools around the country, along with fifty-four lesson plans and teacher training. The cost isn't insignificant—$9,500 per cart—but it's far less expensive than outfitting a classroom with the necessary appliances, and some districts have been able to pay for all or part of the cost with nutrition education grants.

Yet if we're serious about reversing the country's obesity crisis, this can't be an ad hoc effort. If kids don't know how to cook, they'll have no choice as adults but to rely on fast food, restaurant food, and processed food to sustain themselves—an obvious recipe for dietary disaster.

## Growing Good Eating Habits

Gardening is a hands-on form of nutrition education, and programs like Alice Waters's pioneering Edible Schoolyard Project, Slow Food USA's National School Garden Program, and Houston's Recipe for Success all use school gardens to deepen children's understanding of and relationship with food. Studies show they can also make a difference in their eating habits.

For example, since 2010, an organization called FoodCorps has been "embedding" AmeriCorps volunteers in high-need schools to plant gardens and provide experiential learning, like cooking demos and food sampling using the garden-grown food, to change kids' attitudes about healthy eating. According to a 2017 study by the Tisch Food Center at Teachers College, Columbia University, students who engaged in a higher number of FoodCorps' learning activities were found to be eating triple the fruits and vegetables as compared to students participating in fewer of those activities.

*Waking Up Young Taste Buds*

Children understandably shy away from unfamiliar foods, and their knee-jerk, "Yuck!" reaction to new fruits and vegetables can impede healthier eating. But a thoughtful form of sensory-based food education called Sapere has been shown to help.

"The basic idea is very simple," says the writer Bee Wilson, who co-founded the nonprofit TastEd to bring Sapere instruction to kids in the UK. "We encourage children to use all their senses to engage with food in the hope that it will help a person widen his or her palate. The way I describe it is, it's teaching a child how to eat rather than how to cook." "Sapere" means both "to taste" and "to know" in Latin, and the program goes well beyond just exposing children to foods' flavors. "Putting new food in your mouth can be very scary for a child," Wilson explains. "But it's less scary to smell it or touch it or even listen to it. For example, we might break a stick of crunchy celery next to our ears."

Wilson first learned about Sapere education while researching her book *First Bite: How We Learn to Eat* and is now such an ardent believer, she not only helped start TastEd but also serves as one of the organization's classroom teachers. And she's seen firsthand the difference it can make. "One boy said, 'I've never had a peach but I have had peach-flavored medicine,'" Wilson recalls. "And it made me feel happy and sad at the same time because it reminded me why sensory education is so needed. It's impossible to become someone who loves oranges or broccoli if you don't know what they are and have never tasted them."

Research shows that sensory-based food education does reduce children's fear of new foods while helping to instill preferences for healthier foods and more complex flavors. And a 2018 study from the University of Eastern Finland found that the benefits were more pronounced among children whose mothers had a lower educational background, indicating that the program can help reduce societal inequities in children's food choices.

In France, where the principles behind Sapere education were first put into practice in the 1970s, the instruction is actually paid for by the government and built into children's school curriculum, and the same is now true in Finland, Sweden, Denmark, and the Netherlands. The United States is unlikely to follow suit, but Sapere education can also be privately funded, as is the case with TastEd. (The Sapere organization may be able to offer interested parents and organizations ideas for securing that funding; see the Appendix for more information.)

### *"Inoculating" Kids*

If marketing fruits and veggies is one way to improve children's eating habits, we could also take the opposite tack: "inoculating" them against unhealthy food and beverage marketing by helping them see right through it. Two particular approaches seem especially promising:

The first strategy copies the work of anti-tobacco advocates, who often persuade teens not to smoke by showing them how the tobacco industry tries to manipulate them into addiction. This messaging works because it plays right into adolescents' need for autonomy from adults.

In 2016, researchers from the University of Texas at Austin and the University of Chicago's Booth School of Business applied this same principle to unhealthy food. Five hundred eighth graders were divided into two groups, with the first reading an article about healthy eating and the benefits of choosing fresh foods, while the second read an exposé about how food companies make food more addictive and use misleading health claims in their marketing. As one of the researchers later explained in the press, "We cast the executives behind food marketing as controlling adult authority figures, and framed the avoidance of junk food as a way to rebel against their control."

The next day, the students were asked to choose snacks for a long-planned class celebration. Teens in the second group were 11 percent more likely to forgo at least one unhealthy snack, like cookies or chips, in favor of a healthy snack like fruit or baby carrots, and they were 7 percent more likely to spurn sweetened drinks like soda in favor of water. These percentages may seem small, but the researchers calculated that if that behavior was sustained, it could translate into a student losing about a pound of body fat every six to eight weeks.

"[I]f you can appeal to kids' sense of wanting to not be duped, you empower them to take a stand," one of the study's coauthors told a reporter. I had that same thought back in 2013, which inspired me to create a free rhyming video to help inoculate younger kids—those in pre-K through elementary school. The 12-minute video is called "Mr. Zee's Apple Factory" and tells the story of a manufacturer who hooks a town on his deliciously addictive processed foods until the son of a fruit store owner stands up to him.

"Mr. Zee" is laughably low-budget: I couldn't afford a professional artist so I drew the pictures myself, and I enlisted my husband, kids, friends, and neighbors to provide all the voices. But to my surprise and pleasure, this amateur effort has now been viewed almost 50,000 times on YouTube and it's even listed on some teacher websites as a good free resource for nutrition education. Even better, elementary school teachers from around the country (and as far away as Australia) have emailed to tell me that even the littlest kids do respond to the video's message, with some students actually clapping and cheering when a girl at the end of the story bravely bites into a fresh apple.

Another promising counter-messaging technique relates to the relationship between eating and exercise. The food and beverage industries encourage us to "balance" consumption of their unhealthy products with physical activity, like those stickers on stores' refrigerated cases (created by the soda industry's trade group) telling us to "balance what you eat, drink, and do." The parent company of Taco Bell, Pizza Hut, and KFC similarly asserted in a recent corporate responsibility report, "We believe that all of our food can be part of a balanced lifestyle if eaten in moderation and balanced with exercise." This messaging just sounds like common sense, and it conveniently shifts the blame for weight gain to consumers who don't get enough exercise.

But there's a reason why these industries never reveal exactly *how much* exercise would be needed to achieve that elusive "balance"—and letting kids in on that secret holds real promise as another effective inoculation tool. In 2011, researchers at Johns Hopkins found that when African American teens and tweens saw a sign on their corner store's beverage cooler indicating that it would take fifty minutes of jogging to burn off a 20-ounce sugary drink, they were more likely to avoid soda and buy water. Notably, this messaging was significantly more effective than just providing the drink's calorie count. In a later 2014 study, the same researchers found that telling kids they'd have to walk five miles was even more effective, relatively speaking, than the fifty-minute jogging message. And the improvement in kids' buying habits persisted for several weeks, even after the signs were taken down.

## Wish Three: Clean Up the "Claim Game"

According to one recent poll, 64 percent of Americans feel food labels are sometimes or always misleading, while 82 percent said they'd felt "tricked" by nutrition labeling. In another recent poll, 52 percent of low-income parents said they "have a hard time determining which foods are healthy," citing this as a major obstacle in feeding their children a nutritious diet. Clearly, it's time to help clear up all this industry-created confusion.

### At-a-Glance Nutrition Ratings

One way to help shoppers cut through industry-created noise would be a simple front-of-package coding system to rate a product's overall healthfulness—say, from zero to three stars. And in 2011, the Institute of Medicine actually proposed doing just that. Products like chips and cookies would have to show on their packaging that they earned zero stars, a box of granola bars might merit one star, and a loaf of whole-grain bread could boast all three.

But from the food industry's perspective, this star rating system would make it a little *too* easy for consumers to see right through their misleading nutrition claims. So as soon as the industry sensed the Food and Drug Administration was getting more serious about the idea, it quickly preempted the effort by implementing its own "Facts Up Front":

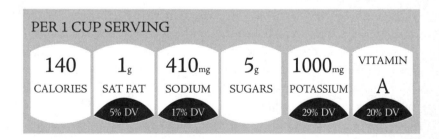

Quick—do those six numbers mean the product is healthy or unhealthy for your kids? Unless you happen to have a calculator handy, it's pretty hard to say. In fact, this "helpful" graphic is so user-*unfriendly* that the Facts Up Front informational website literally greets the visitor with the question, "Wondering what all those numbers are?" In other words: industry mission accomplished.

Instead of labeling that serves industry, we should follow the example of other countries where front-of-package labeling actually serves consumers. In Chile, for example, products too high in sodium, sugar, saturated fat, and/or calories now carry prominent, easily understood black stop signs. And so far, the system appears to be working. Within just one year of the program taking effect, almost 44 percent of Chileans surveyed said they were paying attention to the symbols while shopping; of these, almost 70 percent said they used them to avoid unhealthy products. There are also anecdotal reports of Chilean children being especially aware of the symbols and reminding their parents to heed them in the supermarket. And the new coding system has even nudged manufacturers to reformulate their products: Coca-Cola recently ran a campaign for its new, lower-sugar sodas with a tagline that actually boasted, "Free of Logos [referring to the stop signs], Equally Rich."

Canada, Israel, and Peru are all in the process of developing similar warning-style labeling. Other countries, like the United Kingdom, France, and South Korea, have opted for a red/yellow/green "traffic light" rating system for use on a voluntary basis, while in Ecuador, traffic light ratings recently became mandatory. As in Chile, early data from Ecuador indicates that the color coding is in fact encouraging shoppers to buy healthier products.

Don't American parents deserve this same ability to make quick and informed shopping decisions for their families?

*No More Healthwashing*

Along with a clear front-label coding system, the Food and Drug Administration should also tweak the federal rules to further prevent misleading healthwashing:

+ Products with a disqualifying level of added sugars shouldn't be allowed to make *any* nutrient or health claims. In other words, a sugary cereal shouldn't be able to tout its "whole grain goodness," and Kool-Aid shouldn't be able to claim it's a "good source of vitamin C."

✦ Fruit- or vegetable-related claims (like potato-starch "veggie chips" implying they're chock-full of spinach and tomatoes, or fruit snacks saying they're "made with real fruit") should no longer be allowed if they're based on processed forms of fruits or vegetables, like powders and juice concentrates, which lack the fiber and low-calorie-density that make fresh produce so healthy. The same rule should apply to claims based on other healthy foods, like "yogurt"-covered products that contain only a hint of dried yogurt powder.

✦ Even when a fruit or vegetable claim is based on the use of whole produce, companies should still have to have to say how much and what type of produce is in the product. ("Contains ½ teaspoon of spinach per serving.")

✦ Products like crackers and bread that make a "contains whole grain" claim should also have to disclose the overall percentage or proportion of whole grain, like "15 percent of the grain in this product is whole grain" or "contains 3 grams of whole grain and 17 grams of refined grain."

Just these few simple rule changes would be immeasurably helpful to parents, who too often fall for nutrition claims on products that are, in essence, little better than junk food.

## Wish Four: Improve School Meals

Over 31 million children eat school meals every day and getting those meals right not only improves kids' health, it also shapes their understanding of what a good daily diet looks like. The Healthy, Hunger-Free Kids Act was a huge step forward in school food reform, but too many American kids are still being served a lot of highly processed food in carnival-style menus that only reinforce poor eating habits outside of school.

Here are some ways we could further improve America's school meals:

## Switch Recess

Interestingly, allowing kids to have recess before lunch may make a real nutritional difference. When children aren't chomping at the bit to get outside and play, they're apparently more willing to chomp on fruits and vegetables, as well as drink more milk and waste less food overall. Children who eat lunch after recess also reportedly need less "cool-down" time when they return to the classroom, and one school even saw a 40 percent drop in nurse's visits after it made the switch.

Not all studies have found these benefits, but there's enough anecdotal support for the idea that schools may want to try it out, at least on a pilot basis. (See the Appendix for resources to get started.)

## End School Meal Sugar Overload

School meals currently lack any cap on added sugars—a problem that's especially evident at breakfast, when kids can consume several teaspoons of added sugars at a single meal.

It's a loophole that clearly needs closing, and Margo Wootan, vice president for nutrition at the Center for Science in the Public Interest, believes change is indeed on the horizon. "There will be added sugars standards for school meals in the future," she predicts, "now that there's a specific amount of added sugars recommended in the Dietary Guidelines, and now that all packaged foods will label added sugars." Wootan says the guidelines for Smart Snacks will also need to be revised, "given how weak the total-sugars standard is for many school snacks." (Right now, Smart Snacks items can consist of up to 35 percent sugar by weight.)

## Kick Out the Copycats

The presence of junk-food-branded products in school cafeterias—from Lucky Charms cereal to Doritos tortilla chips—sends kids all the wrong messages about a healthy, daily diet.

That's why we should amend the federal school meal regulations to prevent the offering or sale of any product—even if it meets the Smart Snacks nutrition standards—that's packaged to look just like its unhealthy, off-campus counterpart. In other words, Kellogg's would still be free to sell its whole-grain-rich toaster pastries to schools, but it would no longer be able to brand them as "Pop-Tarts" or use all the same colors and packaging that make kids think they're eating the junk food version sold in supermarkets.

Of course, one reason why companies sell their products to the K-12 market is to get their branding in front of impressionable children on a daily basis. The food and beverage industries would likely push back hard against this proposed regulatory change, but here's some good news: interested school districts can accomplish the same goal through their local school wellness policies. (The Appendix lists resources for crafting this policy language.)

### Give Kids More Time to Eat

Forcing kids to stand in line, get their lunch, and scarf it down all within twenty minutes—common in many districts—can cause real nutritional harm. When kids don't have time to eat their entire meal, fruits and vegetables can be the first foods to wind up in the trash. Children may also eat less food overall, which is especially troubling for the low-income students who rely on school meals for daily nutrition. And too-short lunch periods also deprive kids of the chance to learn how to eat slowly and enjoy food in a social setting.

But it's not just students who bear the brunt of rushed meals. As one school nutrition director complained in an online forum, "When we serve soup, it doesn't cool by the time they have to leave, so it goes into the trash," yet because of food safety regulations "letting it cool off [beforehand] isn't an option." Eat-and-run meals also encourage districts to serve more highly processed hand-held items that can be quickly consumed. And when kids realize they'll get more time to eat if they brown-bag it instead of waiting for a hot meal, families often drop out of the lunch program altogether, drawing needed funds away from the district's food budget.

In overcrowded schools, and particularly those with small cafeterias, there are no easy answers to getting everyone fed in a more leisurely way. But it's also true that school administrators often look to the lunch period first when they need more time for standardized test prep or other instruction. Where there's any room to push back, concerned parents, teachers, and school food directors need to band together and advocate for longer lunch periods.

Here's some food for thought to motivate you: in many other countries, children are given forty-five minutes to an *hour* to eat their meal. Surely we can spare a little more time for the health and well-being of our own kids?

## Help Schools Pay for Labor

School districts in Alaska, Hawaii, and Puerto Rico currently receive extra money from the federal government to compensate for the higher cost of providing school meals in these outlying regions. That makes sense, but it's not as though districts in the forty-eight contiguous states are all operating on the same playing field, either—especially when it comes to hiring labor.

Justin Gagnon's company, Choicelunch, offers healthy meals to private schools and summer camps, as well as some public schools participating in the National School Lunch Program. But because his business is located in Northern California, where labor costs are particularly steep, paying his workers eats up such a large part of the federal reimbursement that it doesn't come close to covering his total per-meal costs. As a result, he can only offer his high-quality meals to the more affluent public schools in his area, ones in which fewer than 10 percent of families rely on the federal subsidy and can instead afford to pay Choicelunch's relatively high lunch fees.

"We need to alter the reimbursement rates to allow for fluctuations in labor costs by metropolitan market," Gagnon suggests, giving districts in areas with high labor costs "a fighting chance at putting more money into their ingredients."

## End the Commodity Program

The National School Lunch Program is run not by the Department of Education, as one might expect, but instead by the Department of Agriculture. And this "strange bedfellows" arrangement produces all kinds of troubling conflicts of interest.

Take Domino's Smart Slice pizza. One of the program's "partners" is the National Dairy Council, which works for Dairy Management Inc., a marketing organization created by the USDA to promote the financial interests of dairy farmers. So even as the USDA tells kids on its My Plate website that pizza should be an "occasional treat," the agency's commodity marketing program is actively pushing Domino's Smart Slice on schools because each slice contains two ounces of cheese—one pound per pie. As one pleased dairy farmer says in a Domino's Smart Slice promotional video, "It's also great for dairymen because as we produce a product, we want to make sure that there's always an outlet for it." Yet that "outlet"—America's school children—already consumes far too much cheese, according to public health experts.

Similarly, the Healthy, Hunger-Free Kids Act regulations originally reflected an Institute of Medicine recommendation that any flavored milk served in schools should be fat-free. But the dairy industry— long alarmed by children's declining milk consumption— successfully lobbied President Trump's USDA in 2018 to ignore that advice and allow not just fat-free flavored milk but also a 1 percent milk-fat variety.

But the most obvious way in which the agricultural industry influences school meals is through the free commodities districts obtain from the federal government, along with their cash reimbursement. This arrangement dates back to the beginning of the National School Lunch Program and reflects the main reason why the federal government became involved in school meals in the first place: to shore up an ailing agriculture sector in the 1930s by finding a use for surplus food. But as we discussed in Chapter 5, about 50 percent of this free commodity food today winds up in the hands of outside processors, which typically turn it into highly processed products like frozen pizza and breakfast pastries. As Boulder's Cooper observes, "The whole lunch program started because we needed to boost farmers, which led us to commodity food, which led us to processed food, which is what sent us down this road."

Indeed, in my informal survey of school nutrition directors, many said they chafed at this longstanding arrangement and wanted more freedom—and more money—in choosing the food they serve kids. As one director—echoed by many others—wrote, "[I wish the USDA would] let schools opt for cash in lieu of commodities, especially since most of the commodities aren't the highest quality." Gagnon wholeheartedly agrees. "I would absolutely do away with commodities, which are a relic of wartime America," he says, "and they keep Big Ag's interest too tightly coupled with the program."

## Tweak the Regulations

As a supporter of the Healthy, Hunger-Free Kids Act, I'm uncomfortable advocating for any loosening of its hard-won nutrition standards. But some progressive school food professionals—the very people trying to feed kids meals that are more nutritious, not less—feel that in an effort to keep a tight grip on potentially irresponsible districts, the government has gone so far in the other direction that sometimes common sense has gone out the window.

"Anytime I'm advocating for loosening regulation," Gagnon says, "I'm sensitive to being lumped in with the people who want to bring back chili cheese fries." But complying with the rules' complex nutrition standards is now so challenging, he says, that running a school meal program is "more of a puzzle than it is a culinary exercise." Boulder's Chef Ann Cooper also feels like something's getting lost in translation. "I do think the nutritional guidelines need to be changed," she says. "They need to be more about food and less about trying to make the numbers balance."

In Gagnon's view, it would be far better to give the good actors more freedom in meal planning and trust that the bad actors will get weeded out. "Ease up on the regulations, and yes, some districts may take advantage of it," he says. "It should be up to the communities—parents, administrators, and school board—to hold their food service operation accountable for delivering a better product, and not a one-size-fits-all set of overly complex regulations at the federal level."

How you feel about Gagnon's suggestion depends on your degree of trust in local communities to do the right thing by kids. I've seen enough blatant disregard for children's health in some districts that I'd rather err on the side of regulatory overkill. Also, the low-income families most dependent on school meals are likely to have the least voice if their district falls down on the job.

Cooper agrees, and would instead focus on tweaking the rules that are already in place. She suggests, for example, fixing current regulatory oddities like having to have two ounces of cheese on each slice of pizza, which she calls "way too much," or having to serve a slice of whole grain bread along with whole grain mac and cheese because the portion size of the entrée isn't quite large enough to meet the grain requirement on its own.

But Cooper wouldn't throw out the baby with the bath water. "I actually think we need the guidelines," she says, "because so many districts would otherwise opt for highly processed, cheaper food."

### Cover the Real Cost of Real Food

In late 2014, the salad chain Sweetgreen posted photos showing typical "School Meals Around the World," in which America's pallid nuggets and canned fruit faced off against gorgeous lunches like Greece's chicken breast on lemon orzo and Spain's grilled shrimp and gazpacho. The photo set turned out to be irresistible click-bait, garnering national media attention and tens of thousands of online views.

What drove me so crazy about the Sweetgreen photos wasn't just their questionable accuracy—Greece doesn't even *have* a school meal program—but the way they subjected America's school food professionals to a huge outpouring of scorn. I can't tell you how many people sent me that link along with some variation of the message: if those other countries can do such a good job, what's wrong with the people running my kid's cafeteria?

But unlike the United States, many countries have venerable, treasured food cultures that both their governments and parents are willing to help preserve by adequately funding school meals. In France, for example, school meal prices are tied to family income and the wealthiest parents can end up paying the equivalent of *seven dollars* or more per meal. In Japan, parents pay around three dollars per meal, but that sum just covers food costs, with the labor and other overhead paid for by the local municipality. (Here in America, districts have to cover their own overhead, leaving just a dollar and change for food.) France and Japan support their meal programs in other ways, too, like generally denying families the ability to send in a packed lunch, so everyone is invested in the same school meal.

America's school meal program was underfunded even before the Healthy, Hunger-Free Kids Act imposed its healthier but often more expensive requirements, and this intense financial pressure encourages schools to sell à la carte "copycat" snacks and offer carnival-style menus just to get kids in the door. Yet if the outsized reaction to the Sweetgreen photos is any guide, many American parents really do want to see something better.

Raising the federal reimbursement rate to meet districts' *actual* needs is the obvious first step toward better school meals. Advocates like Cooper have pegged that rate at around $5 per meal for a student getting a free lunch, which she says would include enough money for healthier food as well as health insurance and a living wage for school food workers. (That's compared to today's $3.46 reimbursement per free lunch, plus the allowance for commodities.) Schools also need additional funding to improve their inadequate kitchens, a nationwide deficit estimated to be $5 billion in 2014.

There's no question this collective price tag would be an exceedingly hard sell in today's political climate. But let's also remember that American parents have never agitated for increased school meal funding in any kind of organized, grassroots way. What if every parent who'd clicked on the Sweetgreen photos turned his or her dissatisfaction into political action during the next Child Nutrition Reauthorization, when Congress funds the school meal program? Would it make a difference if parents joined forces with the School Nutrition Association, perhaps through online petitions, social media, and phone calls to their representatives, to push for a higher reimbursement rate? Maybe not—but we've never tried.

Ultimately, school meal funding comes down to a question of national will. In so many other countries, there's a clear societal willingness to invest in the next generation through healthier, attractive, and delicious school meals. Why not here?

"We need to live in a world," says Cooper, "where we're not spending more on our daily coffee than on school lunch."

### Make Lunch "Free for All"

Now for the most radical proposal: offering school meals to all children, free of charge, regardless of a family's income level.

In my informal survey of school food professionals, a universal meal program was mentioned more often than any other solution to our current school meal problems. First, if meals were free for all students, it would instantly relieve districts of the huge and often quite expensive administrative burden of annually processing all the federal paperwork from families entitled to subsidized meals. All of that money and people-power could instead be focused where it belongs: on preparing healthy food for kids.

Universal meals would also end the stigma currently endured by low-income students, many of whom would rather go hungry than be seen standing in the federally subsidized meal line while their friends get "cool" copycat foods in the à la carte line. Similarly, districts would never again "lunch shame" a child over her unpaid meal balance by having her wear a special wristband or giving her a cold cheese sandwich instead of a hot lunch. Instead, a lunch freely available to all students would become just another integral aspect of the school day, like recess or science class, and it would no longer highlight class distinctions in the cafeteria.

Most importantly, a universal meal program would help alter the current paradigm in which kids are seen as "customers," with all the unhealthy incentives that dynamic creates. Instead of doing their best to mimic off-campus junk food to get kids in the door, schools would feel more freedom to prepare homestyle meals that would not only nourish kids' bodies, but also implicitly teach them what healthier food looks like. The cafeteria could again become a nutrition education classroom, just as many early twentieth century school providers envisioned. As Cooper says, "If school meals were universal, they'd just be seen as part of the educational process of growing the next generation of Americans, and then we'd be looking at this entire issue very, very differently."

So what would it cost to have a universal meal program? In her book *Free for All: Fixing School Food In America*, Janet Poppendieck estimated the additional cost at $12 billion as of 2009. That sounds like a shockingly high figure, and of course it would only be higher today. But by way of comparison, Poppendieck pointed out that $12 billion roughly equaled the cost of just one month of fighting in Iraq and Afghanistan that same year. As for coming up with the funding, Poppendieck walked readers through a number of different ideas, including using the proceeds from a penny-an-ounce federal soda tax to reductions in Farm Bill subsidies for corn and soy.

Unfortunately, the very idea of giving free food to kids who don't need the financial break is anathema to a lot of Americans—despite the fact that we already willingly provide free education to all children, regardless of their family's income. If we ever could muster the necessary political will, however, the funding might well follow. As Poppendieck correctly observed of Congress and its budgetary priorities, "there do seem to be ways of 'finding' money if we really want to."

* * *

I'm aware that many of the proposals I've floated here, particularly those that would most move the needle for children's health, would require federal intervention and, in some cases, a serious outlay of taxpayer dollars. I also know that just talking about these kinds of ideas inevitably attracts heated "nanny state" rhetoric and, often, ugly personal attacks, all of which can make reasoned debate impossible.

Yet every American, regardless of political philosophy, has a vested interest in the health of the next generation. So how did arguably nonpartisan issues like school food and product labeling become so incredibly divisive? And more importantly—for the sake of our children—can we find some common ground?

# 10

# WE'RE BETTER THAN THIS

*I've been focused on starting my kids out with a solid nutritional home life,
which is a huge task, but ... [I now] see we have to change the food
environment for all kids to impact our own.*

~ MOM OF TWO, FAIRFIELD, TEXAS

In January 2015, Texas's newly elected agriculture commissioner, Sid
Miller, held a press conference to announce his first official act in office.
But if Texans expected Miller, a former Republican state lawmaker, to
talk about something related to, well, *agriculture*, they were in for a bit of
a surprise. Instead, Miller stepped up to the podium with a sly grin, held
aloft a frosted pink cupcake, and proclaimed that his first official act
would be "declaring amnesty" for cupcakes in Texas schools.

As Miller explained to the assembled media, a 2004 state school
nutrition policy had banned such treats—"sounds like something from
the Obama administration," he quipped—but in a triumph of "freedom,

liberty, and individual responsibility" over "Big Brother, Big Government control," his office (which oversees federal child nutrition programs in the state) had overturned it. Miller further promised that he would soon overturn the rest of the 2004 policy, which had also prohibited deep-fat fryers and sodas in the state's schools.

The most notable thing about this already notable press conference (held outdoors in front of a Hey Cupcake! food truck, with free cupcakes given to those in attendance) was that there were no existing policies or regulations preventing Texas parents from bringing sugary treats—or any other food, for that matter—to classroom birthday celebrations. To the contrary, Texas has had a state law on its books since 2005 which expressly preserves parents' right to bring to school any food they wish for a child's birthday. This so-called Safe Cupcake Amendment also supersedes any local policies, which means even the most health-conscious Texas district can't override it.

Miller's promised return of sodas and deep-fat fryers was also puzzling. Federal school meal rules (which preempt state regulations) ban all sugar-sweetened sodas on school campuses, and diet sodas can only be sold in high schools. So, at most, Miller's announcement meant Texas high schoolers would soon be able to quaff a Diet Coke—not much of a blow against Big Government. And while Miller could lift the state ban on deep-frying, the majority of districts had abandoned their deep-fat fryers in response to the 2004 policy. In light of the new federal caps on calories and fat in school meals, there was little incentive to go out and buy a new one.

But none of these technicalities mattered to Miller, who likely knew exactly how his seemingly brash policies would be received. They were widely reported in local and national media, including the *Washington Post* and the *Wall Street Journal*, and Miller quickly became the darling of the conservative press. Within just days of taking office, this previously obscure, far-right state politician was chatting with Tucker Carlson on *Fox News* about his commitment to "freedom from burdensome government regulations," while the *National Review* hailed "cupcake amnesty" as "further proof that Texas is the greatest state in the union." A few months later, when Miller did reverse the (diet) soda and (obsolete) fryer bans, he garnered yet more headlines. It all landed Miller squarely on the national map—so much so that he later made the short list to head up President Trump's Department of Agriculture.

And yet . . . as a Texas resident and relatively close observer of the state's school meal program, I don't believe Miller (who won re-election in 2018) is genuinely interested in rolling back school nutrition. Even as his website currently makes the absurd claim that Miller "canceled Michelle Obama's left-wing, feel-good nutrition nonsense that sent more food to the trashcan than to our kids" (last I checked, the U.S. Constitution bars a state official from "canceling" a federal law), in practice, he's done nothing to flout the federal school meal rules or even weaken his department's enforcement of them. To the contrary, he's been a vocal champion of getting more fresh, local produce into schools, and his office awards generous grants—up to $10,000 per school and $50,000 per district— to fund school nutrition education. In other words, Miller might not be Alice Waters, but he's not quite Paula Deen, either.

"Cupcake amnesty" was just a creative spin on an all-too-common tactic: opposing common-sense child nutrition policies for no other reason than ginning up the conservative base. As I mentioned earlier, former New Jersey governor Chris Christie's bashed Michelle Obama's school food reform when it was politically expedient during the 2016 Republican presidential primary, but five years earlier, he'd warmly praised those same efforts. Similarly, Sarah Palin was a notably harsh critic of the former First Lady's anti–childhood obesity campaign, telling conservative radio host Laura Ingraham that she should "leave us alone, get off our back, and allow us as individuals to exercise our own God-given rights to make our own decisions." But as governor of Alaska, Palin had asked for more state funding to combat childhood obesity and also supported a statewide initiative, Living Well Alaska, to improve Alaskans' eating habits.

So how did we get to this unfortunate place, where looking out for kids' health—in the midst of a terrible childhood obesity crisis, no less— has become such a political football?

As a baseline matter, food is an inherently charged issue; our views about food are often shaped by our own upbringing, as well as our race, gender, body image—even religion. We're also experiencing a period of particularly intense food tribalism in this country (among all the other kinds of tribalism that currently divide us), in which proponents of a dietary ideology—veganism, low-carb, paleo, or any other—are often so certain of their views that just talking about food can be a source of friction.

More significantly, though, food is inextricably linked to socioeconomic status. People with fewer resources usually don't have the luxury of carefully considering their food's origins or healthfulness, so when a person seems a little too interested in food, he risks being branded an elitist—and that's especially true in the political sphere. President Martin Van Buren was mocked for hiring a French chef in the White House, while his opponent, William Henry Harrison, was the everyman living on "raw beef and salt." From that 1840 political food smear, we could draw a direct line to a 2004 campaign attack ad calling Howard Dean a "latte-drinking, sushi-eating" liberal, or the glee with which Fox News once pounced on the fact that Barack Obama asked for Grey Poupon on his burger.

On the flip side, chowing down on junk food has become the mark of being a "regular Joe," which is why presidential candidates of both parties feel compelled to eat lots of fried-things-on-a-stick when rubbing elbows with potential voters. When then–Democratic primary candidate John Kerry visited the Iowa state fair in 2003, his press secretary Robert Gibbs was reportedly horrified to see him buying a smoothie. Gibbs was overheard frantically phoning a staffer: "Somebody get a f---ing corn dog in his hand—now!"

And when we're speaking not just about food, but food *policy*, the conversation only becomes more fraught. Debates over food policy typically break along deeply entrenched red/blue lines and, as with so many other political issues, voters sometimes put ideology ahead of their own self-interest. In 2012, the Centers for Disease Control plotted each county's political leaning and its obesity rate on a map, identifying the "Diabetes Belt"—a swath of Southern and Southeastern states where conservative politics and obesity are closely correlated. Perhaps not coincidentally, many of the Diabetes Belt states are the same ones flouting the federal Smart Snacks rules, using a loophole to keep junk food fundraising in their schools.

Much can also depend on the public figures leading these debates. Several recent food policy reforms—from calorie labeling on restaurant menus to the newly improved Nutrition Facts label—were championed by Michelle Obama, which arguably made them even more of a lightning rod for those generally opposed to her husband's administration. Similarly, school food had never been a hugely partisan issue, and it was actually Republican president George W. Bush who laid the groundwork for reform when he directed the Institute of Medicine in 2009 to draft healthier school nutrition standards. Obama was only building on those efforts when she championed the Healthy, Hunger-Free Kids Act, and the law was passed on a bipartisan basis in 2010.

But when control of the House flipped in 2010, that tone shifted. The School Nutrition Association, previously a supporter of the law, now sought to weaken it and found a sympathetic ear among conservative House Republicans. Suddenly, school food was *highly* politicized, and frequently used as a cudgel to bash the Obama administration and the First Lady for their "nanny state" overreach. During that fraught period, I would sometimes wonder what it would have been like if Laura Bush had focused on school food reform instead of literacy as her signature issue. There's no way to know, of course, but it's hard to imagine she'd draw nearly the same kind of fire as Michelle Obama, who endured attacks that *Los Angeles Times* columnist Meghan Daum described at the time as illogical and "astonishingly ugly."

There's also the role of corporate money in our politics. The fast food and restaurant industries are heavily skewed toward the right, historically directing less than 10 percent of their political contributions to Democratic lawmakers. The processed food and beverage industries tend to be more bipartisan in their donations, although they typically step up their contributions to Republicans whenever there's any serious threat of regulation on the horizon. There's nothing wrong with favoring one party over another, of course; what is troubling is the tendency of many conservative lawmakers and pundits to wrap these hugely powerful, multinational corporations in the American flag as they do their bidding, such that any infringement on *their* profit-driven activities somehow becomes an infringement on *your* freedoms as an American citizen.

A perfect example is transparency in nutrition labeling. The improved Nutrition Facts label, its new added sugars disclosure, and calorie labeling in restaurants all came about after hard-fought battles against the food industry. And no wonder: the more we know about some food products, the less likely we may be to buy them. But the industry's allies never own up to what's really at stake: protecting corporate profits. Instead, they make it sound like the mom confused by misleading "fruit" snacks is somehow on the same team as the company intentionally keeping her in the dark. "First Lady Michelle Obama Thinks You're Too Dumb to Read a Nutrition Label," the right-leaning *Washington Examiner* proclaimed, while the then-chairman of the conservative Washington Legal Foundation once argued that clearer product labeling "eat[s] away at consumer freedoms."

Instead of regulation, these critics often make a case for free-market solutions: if enough people want healthier products or clearer labeling, the market will naturally meet consumer demand. But a free market can't function properly if consumers don't have reliable information to make rational purchasing decisions, or if they lack genuine choice in the marketplace.

So long as companies are allowed to make misleading nutrition claims that lend unhealthy products a false health halo, the information provided to consumers is decidedly *un*reliable. And while the 50,000 products in the average supermarket give consumers the illusion of almost infinite choice, just ten powerful multinational corporations— Nestlé, PepsiCo, Coca-Cola, Unilever, Danone, General Mills, Kellogg's, Mars, Associated British Foods, and Mondelez—control almost every major food and beverage brand we buy. This incredible concentration of market power not only limits individual choice, it also gives these corporations outsized influence in our politics, effectively drowning out the voices of ordinary consumers.

All this explains why food policy is generally such a hot-button issue. But when it comes to policies specifically affecting kids, like improving school food, there's another criticism frequently leveled against proposed reforms: that it's the job of parents, not Big Government, to oversee the nutritional quality of children's diets. As Palin put it when criticizing Michelle Obama's anti-childhood obesity efforts, "What she is telling us is she cannot trust parents to make decisions for their own children."

But that argument is a red herring. Even the most left-leaning mom or dad doesn't want a national nanny poking around in their refrigerator or their child's lunch box. Instead, the kinds of policies we're talking about are meant to address relatively recent and harmful shifts in our *external* food environment—changes that have made the job of all parents, regardless of political orientation, exponentially more difficult.

It's also important to note that governmental policies are derided as "nanny state" interventions when they appear to treat adults like children. Yet in the case of policies to improve school meals or ban kid-directed junk food ads, the object of the policy *is* children. And there's nothing remotely new or controversial about using regulations to protect kids' health and safety, such as those relating to age restrictions on the sale of alcohol and tobacco, infant car seats, film and video game ratings, bans on child labor, background checks for childcare workers, and on and on.

Still, any proposal of sweeping policies, even those that would clearly help improve children's health, are almost guaranteed to be met with heated nanny state rhetoric. And, typically, the person making the proposal is also attacked: they might be mocked as a "food fascist," an "anti-pleasure moralist," an "elitist foodie," or the old standard, a "card-carrying member of the Food Police."

That kind of ad hominem nastiness can be hard to brush off, at least for some of us. In fact, almost as soon as I signed the deal with my publisher to write this book, I was paralyzed by anxiety: I could already hear a loud chorus of snide voices calling me just those sorts of names, along with the condescending voices of those who might support some of these proposals in theory, but think it's hopelessly naïve to suggest they could ever become a reality. I just couldn't get this cacophony of anticipated criticism out of my head, and each day I'd stare blankly at my computer, unable to write, and wonder at what point I should start lawyering up for the impending breach of contract litigation with my publisher.

This writer's block sadly persisted not for days or weeks, but for three solid months. Finally, just to feel like I was doing something—anything—to move the project forward, I decided to schedule some interviews with public health experts. I wasn't even looking for quotes at that point, but figured I could at least ask some background questions and that might help get me going.

The first person I contacted was Dr. Shreela Sharma, a professor of epidemiology, human genetics, and environmental sciences at the University of Texas's School of Public Health, and also the co-founder of

Brighter Bites, the nonprofit I mentioned in the last chapter bringing fresh produce to low-income families. Sharma and I had crossed paths in Houston a few times before, and she agreed to meet for breakfast. As we ate, I methodically ran through my list of questions, asking her about everything from population-level nutrient deficiencies to the role of genetics in obesity.

Sharma was so kind and supportive that by the end of the meal, I felt comfortable enough to pour out all the emotional turmoil I'd been feeling about this book. The childhood obesity crisis is so deeply entrenched, I said, and it's going to take dramatic, systemic solutions to reverse course. But our culture has so little tolerance for that kind of intervention, I told her, and it often feels like we can't even have a civil discussion about it. So how can we ever hope to make a real difference in improving children's lives and health?

Sharma paused for a second, then looked me right in the eye and replied in a tone that somehow conveyed both calm certainty and fierce intensity: "We can because we must."

Over the course of the next year, those five words became my mantra. Whenever I felt myself losing the courage of my convictions, I'd remind myself that this is *not a choice*. Our current path is unsustainable, untenable, and, arguably, immoral. The price exacted of our children by today's unhealthy food environment is simply too high.

It was helpful, too, to keep in mind that there are many issues around which even this deeply divided nation should able to find common ground. Every American has a stake in keeping our military strong, for example, which is why 750 retired admirals, generals, and other top military leaders formed a nonpartisan organization in 2010 called Mission: Readiness. Its entire purpose is to sound the alarm over obesity's role in significantly weakening our nation's defense, from the growing number of recruits who are, in its words, "too fat to fight," to an astonishing 72 percent increase in medical evacuations from Iraq and Afghanistan due to injuries typically associated with poor fitness and nutrition.

Then there's the enormous drain on our economy due to obesity, an issue which should allow fiscal conservatives to make common cause with even the most liberal activists. Every obese American incurs an extra $200,000 in direct medical costs over his or her lifetime, and according to a 2016 meta-analysis from the University of Washington, annual medical spending due to obesity was nearly $150 billion—almost enough to fund the entire Department of Veterans Affairs and four times the federal budget for foreign aid. As Dr. David Ludwig has written, "Without obesity, Democrats could conceivably have robust social spending, Republicans could have a balanced budget, and the two parties might find a way to cooperate."

We also need to keep in mind how much progress we've already made. Two decades ago, school hallways were lined with soda machines and many cafeterias were serving kids straight-up junk food. Today, the soda machines are a distant memory and kids are eating more whole grains, fruits, and vegetables in their school meals. Under pressure from health advocates like the Center for Science in the Public Interest, fast food chains are slowly improving their children's menus. And the Walt Disney Company, a huge media conglomerate, no longer allows advertisers to hawk unhealthy foods and drinks to kids on its television channels, radio stations, and websites. These are only a few of the recent developments signaling a positive cultural shift.

Another measure of progress: The Grocery Manufacturers Association, which for decades was a hugely powerful trade group representing all the major food and beverage companies, recently saw its membership dwindle over disagreements about the future of the food industry. While some Big Food behemoths fear change, the corporations that broke ranks clearly believe there's a growing demand for healthier, more transparently labeled products. As Dan Parker, the former food advertising executive, put it to me, "I actually believe that the food industry has already lost this debate. But it's not playing to win, it's playing to lose slowly."

I also take comfort in knowing that American parents, if properly mobilized, are willing to make some noise about these issues. In the Rudd Center for Food Policy & Obesity's 2015 parent survey, 85 percent of parents said companies should reduce their marketing of unhealthy foods and beverages to children. Of these, the vast majority (around 80 percent in each case) said they'd be willing to boycott unhealthy foods that are marketed to children, talk to other parents about the issue, sign an online petition, send an email or letter to a food or beverage company, and send an email or letter to their congressional representative. And those numbers were significantly higher in 2015 than they were in 2012, according to Rudd.

African American and Hispanic parents may be even more willing to engage on these issues, because for many of them it's not just about health but also social justice. In the Rudd survey, parents of color were clearly aware that their children are more aggressively targeted than white children by the food and beverage industries, and they were even more supportive than white parents of a whole host of policies to improve children's food environment. These measures included not just restrictions on advertising but also sugary drink taxes, restricting sugary drink sales near schools, limiting the size of sugary drinks in restaurants, calorie labeling on restaurant menus, and requiring kids' meals with toys to meet certain nutrition standards.

All of this suggests that American parents are a huge source of untapped political power when it comes to enacting measures that would improve kids' health—power that's just waiting to be unleashed with the right messaging at the right time.

And finally, it's reassuring to know that with concerted effort, our culture can shift dramatically in a single generation. When I was a young child in early 1970s, I disliked going to the pediatrician's office, and not just because I dreaded getting a shot. At almost every visit, my pediatrician would light up a cigarette during the appointment, filling the exam room with smoke and filling my nose with his tobacco breath as he leaned in to examine my ears and throat. There's no question in my mind that someday our society will look back on practices like unhealthy children's menus and the aggressive marketing of junk food to children with the same astonishment we'd now feel at the sight of a pediatrician puffing away on a Marlboro.

But that day can't come soon enough. Right now, American children are being shortchanged daily by a diet that feeds but doesn't nourish, that staves off immediate hunger but opens the door to later disease. The factors leading to this tragic outcome are all too human: naked corporate greed; parental ignorance, confusion, and fatigue; practical necessity, for those who can't afford healthier food; and in the case of "treats," even simple love and affection. Improving the current paradigm will require not just pushing back against powerful corporate interests, but also shifting a deeply entrenched food culture.

That's a very heavy lift, but the difficulty of the task doesn't make it any less urgent or critical. And the good news is, there's no shortage of opportunities to pitch in. Whether in corporate boardrooms or kindergarten classrooms, in the halls of Congress or on the sidelines of the soccer field, every one of us has a role to play in forging a brighter, healthier future for the next generation.

We can all do better by our children. We can because we must.

# ACKNOWLEDGMENTS

This book grew out of my blogging at *The Lunch Tray*, so my first thanks must go to my wonderful *Lunch Tray* readership, aka, the "TLT'ers." Without your enthusiastic embrace of the blog, I could never have sustained a near-decade (and counting) of writing about "kids and food, in school and out." Thank you for reading and sharing my posts and for enriching the blog with your own insights and experiences. I'd also like to thank the individual parents who allowed me to interview them here, as well as the hundreds of *Lunch Tray* readers who took the time to respond to my 2018 "Kid Food" survey. Your input was invaluable.

I'm also indebted to Janet Poppendieck, whose excellent book *Free for All: Fixing School Food in America* prompted me to start *The Lunch Tray* in the first place. Thank you, Jan, for empowering me to ask the right questions about school food while instilling empathy for the men and women providing it.

On a related note, I'm grateful to the many school nutrition professionals who've connected with me over the years through my blog, private emails, and the online forum mentioned in Chapter 5. I've learned so much from each of you, and while we sometimes disagree, it's been a particular honor to have earned your trust. Thank you, too, for all your hard work, each and every school day, on behalf of America's most vulnerable kids. I did my best to describe here the many challenges you face, but any inaccuracies in that depiction are my own.

So many other experts generously shared their insights, research, and helpful leads as I wrote *Kid Food*. My gratitude to Helena Bottemiller Evich, Sara Burnett, Beth Collins, Lucy Cooke, Ann Cooper, Carol Danaher, William Dietz, Dan Ellnor, Crystal FitzSimons, Victor Fulgoni III, Justin Gagnon, Josh Golin, Virginia Gray, Andrew Haley, Jennifer Harris, Lisa Helfman, Katie Kattner, Pam Koch, Jim Krieger, Sally Kuzemchak, David Ludwig, Veronica Sau-Wa Mak, Lindsay Moyer, Natalie Digate Muth, Dan Parker, Lindsey Parsons, Claire Raffel, Dina Rose, Lainie Rutkow, Marlene Schwartz, Jeffrey Schwimmer, Shreela Sharma, Michelle Smith, Anneliese Tanner, Henry Voigt, Bee Wilson, and Margo Wootan.

For their research help, thanks to Cheryl Adams and Alison Kelly at the Library of Congress, Jeffrey Boyce at the Child Nutrition Archives of the University of Mississippi's Institute of Child Nutrition, the American Heart Association's Center for Healthy Metrics and Evaluation, and Alex Agboola, formerly at GlobalData.

Thanks to my agent, Elizabeth Kaplan, and to my editor at Oxford University Press, Chad Zimmerman, for believing in this book from the get-go and for patiently fielding my many (*many*) first-time-book-author questions. Thank you, too, Chad, for devoting so much time and attention to *Kid Food* and for being such a pleasure to work with. I'm also grateful to the rest of the Oxford team for making this book a reality, including Sarah Russo, Emily Tobin, Erin Meehan, and Joellyn Ausanka, and to my publicist, Holly Watson.

I can't begin to list all the helpful friends and family members who offered advice or just lent a sympathetic ear as I worked on this project, but I'd feel remiss if I didn't mention Chris Bryan, Dan Elias, Sarah Ellenzweig, Andrew Golub (the first TLT'er), Bronwen Hruska, Lori Lesser, Shirat Mavligit, Scott McGill, Mara Van Nostrand, Dan Oko, and Darcy Pollack. Special thanks to Donna Gershenwald for her always-sage guidance and to Gretchen Debenham Hug for so generously offering her excellent coaching skills when I was hamstrung by writer's block.

I'd also like to take this opportunity to thank some of the many talented women writers who've guided and encouraged me over the years as I aspired to join their ranks: Dana Calvo, Christa Forster, Amy Hertz, Jenny Johnson, Leah Lax, Victoria Ludwin, Samantha Schnee, Andrea White, and Diana Wolfe—and most especially Paula Derrow and Pam

Kaufman, who also served as my readers and first-round editors for *Kid Food*. I'll never be able to adequately thank you, "P & P," not only for helping me find my voice here, but for making me feel safe and supported when I needed it most.

To my wonderful children, Lily and Asher: It was actually the privilege and responsibility of being your mom that first opened my eyes to the many flaws in our food environment, transforming this former Big Food lawyer into a healthy food advocate. But I know it wasn't always easy being my kids, especially back when I was trying to get birthday treats out of your school classrooms or refusing to bring Gatorade to soccer practice like everyone else. (Oh my *god*, Mom!) Thank you for enduring it all with grace and good humor and for putting up with my sorely divided attention as I wrote this book. I'm so proud of the caring, thoughtful young adults you've both become, and I love you more than I can say.

When people learned that my husband, Martin, and I were both at home writing books, their response was usually a pointed question about the square footage of our house or just an open expression of amazement that we hadn't yet killed each other. I never understood those reactions, though, because I can't think of anyone with whom I'd rather share my day than you, "Mr. TLT." Your sharp intellect always inspires me to think more critically, you never fail to make me laugh, and even though it took time away from our family life, produced negligible income, and at one point even brought a subpoena to our door, you've never once wavered in your support of my writing and advocacy. Truly, no one could ask for a better partner in love and life.

Finally, my gratitude to two women who, each in her own way, indelibly shaped me and therefore this book: Dana Woldow, of blessed memory, for her warm friendship, invaluable mentorship, and decades of selfless advocacy to give all children access to healthier school food without shame or stigma; and most especially, Midge Elias, whose caring commitment to feeding her own kids healthfully laid the foundation for my interest in this topic, and whose unqualified love and support have buoyed me throughout my life.

I love you, Mom—and I'm sorry for making fun of your oatmeal "cookies."

# APPENDIX

Here are some of my favorite books, websites, and other resources addressing many of the topics covered in *Kid Food*.

## Help with Child Feeding and Picky Eating

### Books

There are many books purporting to "fix" your child's picky eating, but as we know, picky eating isn't necessarily a "problem" and "fixing" it can do more harm than good. I especially like these books for their sound approach:

*Child of Mine: Feeding with Love and Good Sense,* by Ellyn Satter. Written by the well-known expert who originated the Division of Responsibility model we discussed in Chapter 2, this book is widely considered the bible of infant and child feeding.

*It's Not About the Broccoli: Three Habits to Teach Your Kids for a Lifetime of Healthy Eating,* by Dina Rose. A sociologist and child feeding expert asks parents to think less about the specific foods their kids are eating (or not eating) and focus instead on the life-long eating habits parents hope to instill.

*Stress-Free Feeding: How to Develop Healthy Eating Habits in Your Child,* by Lucy Cooke and Laura Webber. An accessible and practical guide to feeding children from infancy through age five, including how to navigate various feeding problems as they crop up.

*"Eat Your Vegetables" and Other Mistakes Parents Make: Redefining How to Raise Healthy Eaters,* by Natalie Digate Muth. A pediatrician, registered dietitian, and mom of two examines twelve common feeding mistakes, from "Forbidding Potato Chips and Ice Cream" to "Catering to Picky Eaters." Each chapter thoughtfully examines why parents make these mistakes, then offers counterstrategies to help them reverse course.

*The Picky Eater Project: 6 Weeks to Happier, Healthier Family Mealtimes,* by Natalie Digate Muth and Sally Sampson. A six-week plan to address picky eating, mainly by involving kids in grocery shopping and cooking. It offers a trove of recipes, feeding advice, shopping tips, kids' kitchen projects, and more.

*Fearless Feeding: How to Raise Healthy Eaters from High Chair to High School,* by Jill Castle and Maryann Jacobsen. Two registered dietitians join forces to calm and empower parents by offering step-by-step feeding advice for every developmental stage. A revised and updated edition was released in 2019.

*From Picky to Powerful: The Mindset, Strategies and Know-How You Need to Empower Your Picky Eater,* by Maryann Jacobsen. By explaining how and why picky behaviors crop up, as well as the importance of respecting kids' individual differences, Jacobsen helps parents figure out when to worry and when to let go.

*Helping Your Child With Extreme Picky Eating: A Step-By-Step Guide For Overcoming Selective Eating, Food Aversion, and Feeding Disorders,* by Katja Rowell and Jenny McGothlin. A remarkably comprehensive and compassionate resource for families grappling with more extreme forms of picky eating, including ARFID (Avoidant Restrictive Food Intake Disorder.)

*French Kids Eat Everything: How Our Family Moved to France, Cured Picky Eating, Banned Snacking, and Discovered 10 Simple Rules for Raising Happy, Healthy Eaters,* by Karen Le Billon. In this entertaining memoir, Le Billon, a Canadian, describes the year she spent in her French husband's small hometown, during which their two young daughters gradually abandoned their picky ways. In a follow-up book, *Getting to Yum: The 7 Secrets of Raising Eager Eaters,* Le Billon distills the feeding advice she gleaned from living in France.

*First Bite: How We Learn to Eat,* by Bee Wilson. A fascinating exploration of how people form their taste preferences. Though not an advice or child feeding book, *First Bite* may well change how parents view their children's eating habits—and their own.

## Blogs and Websites

Here are some of my favorite blogs and websites relating to child feeding and picky eating, some of which belong to authors mentioned above.

*Real Mom Nutrition*
*Raise Healthy Eaters*
*The Nourished Child*
*Extreme Picky Eating*

## Help with Family Dinner: Recipes, Tips, and More

All cookbooks offer recipes, of course, but not all of those recipes hit the tasty/healthy/fast sweet spot that's so critical on busy weeknights. Here are some cookbooks, websites, and blogs that make the cut:

## Books

**Cooking Light** *Dinnertime Survival Guide: Feed Your Family, Save Your Sanity,* by Sally Kuzemchak. This book lives up to its promise of helping parents overcome just about any obstacle getting in the way of family dinner. On a tight food budget? No clue how to cook? Can't get everyone to the table at the same time? Dietitian and mom Kuzemchak not only has the answers, she serves them up with healthy, kid-approved recipes.

*Dinner: A Love Story—It All Begins at the Family Table,* by Jenny Rosenstrach. Based on Rosenstrach's blog of the same name, *Dinner: A Love Story* is both memoir and cookbook, and it will keep weeknight chefs inspired with delicious but doable recipes.

*The Six o'Clock Scramble: Quick, Healthy, and Delicious Dinner Recipes for Busy Families* and *SOS! The Six o'Clock Scramble to the Rescue: Earth-Friendly, Kid-Pleasing Dinners for Busy Families*, by Aviva Goldfarb. Every busy parent dreads that moment at six o'clock when a hungry family asks, "What's for dinner?" These two cookbooks offer pared-down recipes, many of which can be prepared in as little as half an hour.

*100 Days of Real Food: How We Did It, What We Learned, and 100 Easy, Wholesome Recipes Your Family Will Love*, by Lisa Leake. After cutting out all processed food for one hundred days, Leake's family never looked back. This cookbook shares their story along with shopping tips and easy, real-food recipes.

### Blogs and Websites

Here are some of my favorite blogs and websites offering family dinner help, some of which belong to authors mentioned above.

*Smitten Kitchen (Weeknight Favorites)*
*New York Times Cooking (Easy Weeknight Recipes)*
*Food Network (Family-Friendly Weeknight Dinner Recipes)*
*Dinner: A Love Story*
*Simply Recipes*
*Mom's Kitchen Handbook*
*100 Days of Real Food*
*Real Mom Nutrition*

### Cookbooks for Kids

Teaching your child how to cook is a gift that will pay a lifetime of dividends. Here are a few of my favorite cookbooks just for kids:

*Complete Children's Cookbook* (**DK**). A straightforward and well-photographed cookbook to teach kids aged seven to ten how to make more than 150 basic recipes, from French toast to lasagna.

*Eat Your Greens, Reds, Yellows, and Purples: Children's Cookbook* (**DK**). Designed for children aged eight to twelve, this colorful vegetarian cookbook offers twenty-five recipes centered around fruits and vegetables.

*Chop Chop.* Not a book but a quarterly magazine, *Chop Chop* is published in both Spanish and English and filled with nutritious, ethnically diverse, and inexpensive recipes just for kids. It also has fun food facts, games, puzzles, and interviews. Subscribe at http://www.chopchopmag.org/.

*Favorites for New Cooks: 50 Delicious Recipes for Kids to Make,* by Caroline Federman. A lovely children's cookbook written by the cofounder of the Charlie Cart Project, which brings home economics back to schools through mobile kitchens. In addition to its healthy recipes, the book includes some fun kitchen science and food history.

*Pretend Soup and Other Real Recipes: A Cookbook for Preschoolers and Up,* by Mollie Katzen and Ann Henderson. Coauthored by Katzen, the renowned *Moosewood* chef, this popular cookbook teaches cooking skills and food literacy to children as young as three and up to age eight.

*The Picky Eater Project: 6 Weeks to Happier, Healthier Family Mealtimes,* by Natalie Digate Muth and Sally Sampson. Not only for picky eaters, this book offers a trove of recipes and kitchen projects just for young chefs.

*A Smart Girl's Guide: Cooking: How to Make Food for Your Friends, Your Family & Yourself,* by Patricia Daniels and Darcie Johnston. Part of the popular American Girl Smart Girl's Guides series, this book for young and tween girls takes a breezy, accessible approach to cooking.

*The Complete Cookbook for Young Chefs,* by America's Test Kitchen Kids. In an accessible format that never talks down to its young readership, this cookbook offers simple, approachable recipes that were reportedly tested by more than 750 kids.

*The Young Chef: Recipes and Techniques for Kids Who Love to Cook,* by the Culinary Institute of America. Kids aged ten to fourteen can learn from the country's most prestigious culinary school via this popular cookbook. After teaching kids some basic techniques and kitchen lingo, it offers over one hundred recipes to let them explore their creativity in the kitchen.

*The Little House Cookbook: New Full-Color Edition: Frontier Foods from Laura Ingalls Wilder's Classic Stories,* by Barbara M. Walker. For young fans of the Little House books, this award-winning cookbook recreates more than one hundred of the foods mentioned by Laura Ingalls Wilder in her stories—everything from corn dodgers to vanity cakes. The cookbook was first published in 1979 and was re-released in 2018 in a new format with color photographs.

## Teaching Kids Food Literacy

Here are a few of my favorite resources to teach your kids more about food and where it comes from:

*Starting with Soil,* from the Center for Ecoliteracy. This free tablet app features gorgeous photography and an interactive interface to teach children aged six to twelve about how soil is formed, the roles animals and people play in keeping it healthy and fertile, and the basics of seeds, pollinators, and organic farming practices.

*The 101 Healthiest Foods for Kids: Eat the Best, Feel the Greatest—Healthy Foods for Kids and Recipes Too!* by Sally Kuzemchak. A family-friendly guide to help kids (and adults) explore new and nutritious foods—everything from farro to papayas. Packed with recipes, nutrition information, tips, and more.

**Readers to Eaters** is a publishing company founded in 2009 exclusively to help promote children's food literacy. It features an ever-growing number of titles meant to give kids and families a better understanding of "what and how we eat." http://www.readerstoeaters .com/our-books/.

*Eating the Alphabet,* by Lois Ehlert. A beloved and beautiful board book that teaches the youngest eaters about fruits and vegetables, from A to Z.

*Eat Up! An Infographic Exploration of Food,* by Antonia Banyard and Paula Ayer. A colorful infographic book for tweens to help them better understand our food system.

# Food Politics for Kids

Here are some resources to teach older children about our food system and the various forces that shape it:

*Chew on This: Everything You Don't Want to Know About Fast Food,* by Eric Schlosser and Charles Wilson. For kids twelve and older, a teen-oriented version of Schlosser's groundbreaking 2001 book, *Fast Food Nation.*

*The Omnivore's Dilemma: Young Reader's Edition,* by Michael Pollan. Pollan's classic 2007 book, edited for kids aged ten and up.

**In Defense of Food,** a free curriculum for kids aged ten to fourteen, developed by the Tisch Food Center at Teachers College, Columbia University. It serves as a companion for the PBS series based on Michael Pollan's 2008 book of the same name, and covers a wide range of food-related topics.

*What's on Your Plate?* This 2009 documentary directed by Catherine Gund follows two eleven-year-old New York City girls as they examine the various food systems in their city and its surroundings.

## Teaching Kids to see through Food Marketing

*Eat This! How Fast Food Marketing Gets You to Buy Junk (and How to Fight Back)* by Andrea Curtis. A terrific book designed to teach kids aged nine to twelve about food and beverage marketing, including the tools they need to help decode it.

*Mr. Zee's Apple Factory,* by Bettina Elias Siegel. Here's a little plug for my own free, twelve-minute video for younger kids. It's an illustrated, rhyming story of a food manufacturer who hooks an unsuspecting town on processed food—until the son of a fruit store owner fights back. https://www.youtube.com/watch?v=xEN4UTbovKM.

## Cooking And Taste Education

Here's information on two particularly promising food education programs mentioned in *Kid Food*:

The Charlie Cart Project brings mobile, compact kitchens to interested schools, along with an integrated educational program that connects food and cooking to other academic subjects. www.charliecart.org.

Sapere is the international nonprofit devoted to providing taste education for children at school. For information on starting Sapere instruction in your area, visit http://sapere-asso.fr/en/contact/.

## General Resources for Parent Advocates

Here are of some of my favorite organizations offering general information and guidance for aspiring parent food advocates:

UConn Rudd Center for Food Policy & Obesity
Center for Science in the Public Interest
Voices for Healthy Kids
Action for Healthy Kids
Parents for Healthy Kids
Alliance for a Healthier Generation
Chef Ann Foundation
The Edible Schoolyard Project

## Addressing the Junk Food in your Child's Daily Life

So much of the unhealthy food in our kids' lives comes in the form of snacks and "treats" at daily activities. Here are two resources to help push back:

*The Snacktivist's Handbook,* by Sally Kuzemchak. A useful guide to improving the snacks offered in youth sports, camps, schools, and more. Includes research-backed information, advocacy tips, and even sample letters you can send to your team coach and other treat-doling adults. Available for purchase at the *Real Mom Nutrition* blog, https://www.realmomnutrition.com/snacktivists-handbook/.

*The Lunch Tray's Guide to Getting Junk Food Out of Your Child's Classroom* (2nd edition), by Bettina Elias Siegel. My free, 50-page e-book devoted specifically to cleaning up the unhealthy food

offered in school classrooms. Sign up for your free copy at www.
thelunchtray.com/free-guide/.

## Information on Kids and Sugar

Because sugary foods and drinks are offered to kids in so many contexts,
it's useful to be armed with the latest scientific guidance:

"Kids and Added Sugars: How Much Is Too Much?" American
Heart Association, https://www.heart.org/en/news/2018/
05/01/kids-and-added-sugars-how-much-is-too-much.
"Sugar Recommendation Healthy Kids and Teens Infographic,"
American Heart Association, http://www.heart.org/en/healthy-
living/healthy-eating/eat-smart/sugar/sugar-recommendation-
healthy-kids-and-teens-infographic.
*The Lunch Tray's Guide to Getting Junk Food Out of Your Child's
Classroom* (2nd edition) My free 50-page e-book includes a general discussion about kids and sugar. Sign up at www.thelunchtray.
com/free-guide/.

## School Food Reform

Nothing will earn your school nutrition director's trust more than showing you did your homework before asking for changes to school meals.
Here are resources to help learn how the federal meal program works—
and how to make it better:

### Books

*Free for All: Fixing School Food in America,* by Janet Poppendieck.
Though written shortly before school meals were overhauled by
the Healthy, Hunger-Free Kids Act, *Free for All* still provides an
excellent education on the federal school meal program's evolution from an anti-hunger initiative in the 1940s to the flawed
program we have today.
*School Lunch Politics: The Surprising History of America's Favorite
Welfare Program,* by Susan Levine. Another informative and

entertaining history of the program, for those who want to take a deep dive.

## Blogs and Websites

**Dana Woldow's writings (PEACHSF), archived on *The Lunch Tray*.** For over twenty years, the late Dana Woldow worked tirelessly as an advocate for better school food in her local San Francisco district and nationally. She generously wrote up everything she'd learned along the way in easy-to-read, concise essays, like "Everybody's Guide to Fixing School Food," and "How to Make Friends with Your Nutrition Services Director." Before her death in 2017, Woldow's materials were housed on her own website, PEACHSF (Parents, Educators & Advocates Connection for Healthy School Food). I'm now honored to be the curator of this invaluable material, which is archived under its own PEACHSF link on *The Lunch Tray*. More than any other resource, I recommend that novice school food reformers start here. https://thelunchtray.com/peachsf-resources-for-school-food-advocacy.

**The Food and Nutrition Service** of the U.S. Department of Agriculture oversees all federal childhood nutrition programs, including school meals. The FNS website has facts and figures about the program, nutrition standards, reimbursement rates, annual participation data and more. https://www.fns.usda.gov/nslp/national-school-lunch-program-nslp.

**The School Nutrition Association** is the group that represents 58,000 school food professionals. While the organization's website is geared toward its members, it contains useful information for parents interested in learning more about school meals. www.schoolnutrition.org.

**Chef Ann Foundation's "Parent Advocacy Toolkit"** offers a range of resources from Chef Ann Cooper's foundation, including information on grants for salad bars and school gardens, guidance on forming coalitions, even model answers to the arguments you're most likely to encounter from resistant decision makers. http://www.chefannfoundation.org/for-parents/parent-advocacy-toolkit/.

UConn Rudd Center for Food Policy & Obesity "School Food Landscape" offers a wealth of information, resources, and advice for parents trying to improve school food. http://www.uconnruddcenter.org/food-landscape.

"No- or Low-Cost Policies to Support a Healthy School Nutrition Environment," Center for Science in the Public Interest. Though written for school food professionals, parents can learn a lot from this two-pager. https://cspinet.org/sites/default/files/attachment/School-Meals-Tip-Sheet-No-or-Low-Cost-Policies.pdf.

"Eat Better in the Cafeteria," Action for Healthy Kids. Ideas for helping students eat more healthfully in the cafeteria. http://www.actionforhealthykids.org/game-on/find-challenges/cafeteria-challenges#cafeteria.

"School Meals," an overview from the Centers for Disease Control and Prevention, https://www.cdc.gov/healthyschools/npao/schoolmeals.htm.

## Farm-to-School Resources

For parents and school food professionals interested in learning more about bringing local produce to their school cafeterias:

National Farm-to-School Network, http://www.farmtoschool.org/.

"Starting a Farm-to-School Program," KidsHealth, https://kidshealth.org/en/parents/farm-to-school.html/.

"Farm-to-School Resources for Parents," Georgia Organics, https://georgiaorganics.org/for-schools/the-farm-to-school-resources-for-parents/.

## Tips on Scheduling Recess before Lunch

Making the switch is sometimes easier said than done. Here's help:

"Benefits of Recess Before Lunch Fact Sheet," Peaceful Playgrounds, https://www.peacefulplaygrounds.com/download/lunch/benefits-recess-before-lunch-facts.pdf.

"Recess Before Lunch: Optimizing School Schedules to Support Learning," Montana Team Nutrition, http://www.nea.org/archive/43158.htm.

"Recess Before Lunch," Action for Healthy Kids, http://www.actionforhealthykids.org/tools-for-schools/find-challenges/cafeteria-challenges/1232-recess-before-lunch.

## Wellness Policies

Here are resources to help you understand what wellness policies do, how to draft one, how to evaluate its strength, and how to implement it:

"Local School Wellness Policy," U.S. Department of Agriculture, Food and Nutrition Service. Here you'll find links to the federal rule governing wellness policies, along with other tools, FAQs, and more. https://www.fns.usda.gov/tn/local-school-wellness-policy.

"School Nutrition Environment and Wellness Resources," U.S. Department of Agriculture, Food and Nutrition Service. An even more comprehensive page from the USDA, with additional information relating to the drafting and implementation of wellness policies. https://healthymeals.fns.usda.gov/local-wellness-policy-resources/school-nutrition-environment-and-wellness-resources/site-map.

School Wellness Policies.org, a website devoted to explaining wellness policies to parents, created by the National Alliance for Nutrition and Activity. http://www.schoolwellnesspolicies.org/.

WellSAT 3.0, the Wellness School Assessment Tool was created by the UConn Rudd Center for Food Policy & Obesity and can be used by districts and parents to first score and then strengthen their existing wellness policy. http://www.wellsat.org/.

"School Wellness Policies 101," Action for Healthy Kids, http://www.actionforhealthykids.org/storage/documents/parent-toolkit/parent-leadership-series/wellnesspolicyvfinalx.pdf.

Local School Wellness Policy, Centers for Disease Control and Prevention. A basic overview of wellness policies, with additional links. https://www.cdc.gov/healthyschools/npao/wellness.htm.

*The Lunch Tray's Guide to Getting Junk Food Out of Your Child's Classroom* (2nd edition). My free 50-page e-book includes a general discussion of wellness policies, among other resources. Sign up at www.thelunchtray.com/free-guide/.

## Ending Classroom Food Rewards

When asking teachers or schools to stop using food rewards, it's helpful to have the latest research on why the practice is a bad idea, as well as ideas for non-food alternatives:

"White Paper: The Use of Food as a Reward in Classrooms: The Disadvantages and the Alternatives," by Alicia Fedewa, Anita Courtney, and Casey Hinds. In gathering relevant research counseling against the use of food rewards, this document is invaluable for parent advocates. https://kyhealthykids.files.wordpress.com/2014/04/whitepaper.pdf.

*The Lunch Tray's Guide to Getting Junk Food Out of Your Child's Classroom* (2nd edition), by Bettina Elias Siegel. My free 50-page e-book has a section on classroom food rewards. Sign up at www.thelunchtray.com/free-guide/.

"Food as a Reward," UConn Rudd Center for Food Policy & Obesity. http://ruddroots-dev.port200.com/school-food/food-outside-the-cafeteria/food-as-a-reward.

"Constructive Classroom Rewards Fact Sheet," Center for Science in the Public Interest. https://cspinet.org/resource/constructive-classroom-rewards-fact-sheet.

## Getting Copycat Products and other Junk Food Marketing out of Schools

Though this topic is generally covered in the resources for wellness policies, here are some materials specifically addressing food and beverage marketing in schools, including the sale of junk food-branded products in the cafeteria:

"'Look-alike' Smart Snacks in Schools," UConn Rudd Center for Food Policy & Obesity. This page provides links to the latest research on copycat products, videos and presentations for advocates, fact sheets, and more. http://uconnruddcenter.org/lookalikesmartsnacks.

"Restricting Food and Beverage Marketing in Schools," ChangeLab Solutions. A useful four-page document on why this marketing should be limited and how to do it. https://www.changelabsolutions.org/sites/default/files/Restricting_Food_and_Beverage_Marketing_in_Schools-FINAL-201705.pdf.

"Food and Beverage Marketing: Model School Wellness Policy Language," ChangeLab Solutions. Guidance on including a provision in your district's local school wellness policy to ban copycat products. https://www.changelabsolutions.org/sites/default/files/ModelLocalSchoolWellnessPolicyLanguage_FINAL_201705_0.pdf.

"Local Wellness Policies and Junk Food Marketing Fact Sheet," Voices for Healthy Kids, https://schoolwellness.voicesforhealthykids.org/resources/local-wellness-policies-and-junk-food-marketing-fact-sheet/.

### Healthier School Fundraising

Junk food fundraisers are easy, but healthy fundraising doesn't have to be hard. Here's help:

"Healthy Fundraisers," Action for Healthy Kids, http://www.actionforhealthykids.org/storage/documents/pdfs/tipsheets-may-2018/fundraisers-family-health-8-6-17.pdf.

"Best Practices for Healthy School Fundraisers," U.S. Department of Agriculture, Food and Nutrition Service, https://www.fns.usda.gov/best-practices-healthy-school-fundraisers.

"Promote Good Health While Raising Money for Schools," Pew Charitable Trusts, https://www.pewtrusts.org/en/research-and-analysis/articles/2015/08/13/promote-good-health-while-raising-money-for-schools.

# Healthier Classroom Parties

Classroom parties don't have to be a cake-and-soda fest. Here are fun, creative, and easy ideas for healthier school parties:

*The Lunch Tray's Guide to Getting Junk Food Out of Your Child's Classroom* (2nd edition), by Bettina Elias Siegel. Sign up for my free 50-page e-book at www.thelunchtray.com/free-guide/.

*The Lunch Tray's* Pinterest boards offer a wealth of ideas for healthy classroom parties for students' birthdays, Valentine's Day, Halloween, and more. www.pinterest.com/thelunchtray.

"Healthy and Active Classroom Parties," Action for Healthy Kids, http://www.actionforhealthykids.org/tools-for-schools/1249-healthy-and-active-classroom-parties.

"Healthy School Celebrations," Center for Science in the Public Interest, https://cspinet.org/resource/healthy-school-celebrations.

# NOTES

## Front Matter

ix   *frozen fruit, bagged salad greens, and baby carrots are all "processed" foods* International Food Information Council, "What Is Processed Food? You Might Be Surprised!" https:// foodinsight.org/wp-content/uploads/2014/07/IFIC_ Handout1_high_res.pdf; Jenny Splitter, "'Processed Food' Gets an Unfair Bad Rap," *New York*, October 10, 2017, https://www .thecut.com/2017/10/processed-food-gets-an-unfair-bad-rap .html?utm_source=tw&utm_medium=s3&utm_campaign =sharebutton-b.

ix   *when preparing and preserving food was an exhausting, full-time endeavor* See, e.g., Rachel Laudan, "In Praise of Fast Food," *Utne Reader*, September and October, 2010, https://www.utne.com/ Environment/Fast-Food-Culinary-Ethos.

x    **Betty Crocker Blastin' Berry Hot Colors Fruit Roll-Ups** Ingredient listing found at https://www.bettycrocker.com/products /fruit-snacks/fruit-roll-ups/fruit-roll-ups-blastin-berry-hot -colors.

x    *a classification system called "NOVA"* Monteiro and his team have published many articles over the years about the NOVA system, but my discussion here is based on Carlos A. Monteiro et al., "Food Classification. Public Health NOVA. The Star Shines Bright," *World Nutrition* 7, nos. 1–3 (January–March 2016).

x    *description of the other three categories [of the NOVA system]* The other three NOVA classifications are: *Group One— Unprocessed or Minimally Processed Foods*, which includes: fresh, dried, or frozen fruits and vegetables; grains and legumes; pasta; whole grain flours; eggs; fresh or frozen meats and fish; and milk. *Group Two—Processed Culinary Ingredients*, which includes: sugar, oils, salt, and other substances extracted from foods or nature, and which are used to season or cook. These foods are rarely eaten alone. *Group Three—Processed Foods*, which are relatively simple products, usually with just a few ingredients, that are made by adding substances in Group Two to the foods in Group One. Examples include: vegetables in brine; fruits in syrup; salted meats and fish; salted or sugared nuts and seeds; cheese; and freshly made, unpackaged breads.

xi    *so pleasurable that some experts believe they're actually addictive* See, e.g., David A Kessler, *The End of Overeating: Taking Control of the Insatiable American Appetite* (New York: Rodale, 2010).

xi    *"Eat all the junk food you want as long as you cook it yourself"* Michael Pollan, *Food Rules: An Eater's Manual* (New York: Penguin, 2009), 85.

xi    *Some people have criticized the NOVA system* Critiques of the NOVA classifications include: Michael J. Gibney et al., "Ultra-Processed Foods In Human Health: A Critical Appraisal," *American Journal of Clinical Nutrition* (September 2017), doi:10.3945/ajcn.117.160440; Anthony Warner, *Angry Chef* blog, "Rise of the Ultra Foods—Part 1," April 2, 2018, angry-chef.com/blog/rise-of-the-ultra-foods-part-1 and "Rise of the Ultra Foods—Part 2," April 14, 2018, angry-chef.com/blog/rise-of-the-ultra-foods-part-2.

xi    *Correlation between a diet high in ultra-processed food and serious health concerns* A number of recent studies have established a clear correlation between a diet high in ultra-processed foods and an increased risk of certain diseases as well as overall mortality. See Bernard Srour et al., "Ultra-processed Food Intake and Risk of Cardiovascular Disease: Prospective Cohort Study (NutriNet-Santé)," *BMJ*, (2019): L1451, doi:10.1136/bmj.l1451 (a 10 percent increase in the proportion of ultra-processed foods in the diet was associated with a 10 percent increased risk of cardiovascular diseases); Thibault Fiolet et al., "Consumption of Ultra-processed Foods and Cancer Risk: Results from NutriNet-Santé Prospective Cohort." *BMJ* (2018): 360:k322, doi:10.1136/bmj.k322 (a 10 percent increase in the proportion of ultra-processed foods in the diet was associated with a 12 percent increased risk of cancer); Laure Schnabel et al., "Association Between Ultraprocessed Food Consumption and Risk of Mortality Among Middle-aged Adults in France," *JAMA Internal Medicine* 179, no. 4 (2019): 490, doi:10.1001/jamainternmed.2018.7289 (a 10 percent increase in the consumption of ultra-processed foods was correlated with a 15 percent increase in all-cause mortality); Anaïs Rico-Campà et al., "Association between Consumption of Ultra-processed Foods and All Cause Mortality: SUN Prospective Cohort Study," *BMJ* (2019): L1949, doi:10.1136/bmj.l1949 (more than 4 daily servings of ultra-processed food correlated with a 62 percent increased risk of all-cause mortality; each serving of ultra-processed food raised the risk of dying by 18 percent.) A 2019 study also found that when subjects were offered a diet consisting mostly of ultra-processed foods and beverages, they consumed, on average, an additional 500 calories per day as compared to their intake when offered a diet rich in whole foods. Kevin D. Hall et al., "Ultra-processed Diets Cause Excess Calorie Intake and Weight Gain: A One-month Inpatient Randomized Controlled Trial of Ad Libitum Food Intake," *Cell Metabolism* (2019), doi:10.31232/osf.io/w3zh2.

## Introduction

4    *and reading this book*—**Free for All: Fixing School Food in America** Janet Poppendieck, *Free for All: Fixing School Food in America* (Berkeley: University of California Press, 2010).

10 *I willingly shared my best advice* My 50-page ebook, *The Lunch Tray's Guide to Getting Junk Food Out of Your Child's Classroom*, is available for free download at http://www.thelunchtray.com/free-guide/.

12 *other mothers may accuse you of negligence* Tony Posnanski, "Feeding My Kids Processed Foods Is Not Child Abuse," *Huffington Post*, April 28, 2014, https://www.huffingtonpost.com/tony-posnanski/feeding-my-kids-processed-foods-is-not-child-abuse_b_5143063.html.

12 *you might be called a gullible alarmist...or...a "sancti-mommy"* Jenny Splitter, "Stop Telling Me I'm Poisoning My Kids: Food Crusaders, Sancti-Mommies and the Rise of Entitled Eaters," *Salon*, December 8, 2015, https://www.salon.com/2015/12/05/stop_telling_me_im_poisoning_my_kids_food_crusaders_sancti_mommies_and_the_rise_of_entitled_eaters/.

13 *a carefree embrace of junk food is a sign of being a "real" American* See, e.g., Jane Black and Brent Cunningham, "Next Up In the Culture Wars: Food Fights," *Washington Post*, November 27, 2010, http://www.washingtonpost.com/wp-dyn/content/article/2010/11/26/AR2010112603494.html; Kristin Wartman, "The American Fast Food Syndrome," *Civil Eats*, January 12, 2011, https://civileats.com/2011/01/13/the-american-fast-food-syndrome/.

13 *politicians...chow down on junk food or fast food while the cameras are rolling* Katie Zezima, "Obama Tries To Connect With Ordinary Americans—Through Junk Food," *Washington Post*, July 18, 2014, https://www.washingtonpost.com/news/post-politics/wp/2014/07/18/obama-tries-to-connect-with-ordinary-americans-through-junk-food/?utm_term=.b0c51007557e; Maxwell Tani, "Here Are the Best Pictures of the Presidential Candidates Eating Greasy, Fried Food at Iowa State Fair," *Connecticut Post*, August 19, 2015, https://www.ctpost.com/technology/businessinsider/article/Here-s-all-the-greasy-fatty-fried-food-6446286.php.

13 *former New Jersey governor Chris Christie* Bettina Elias Siegel, "Christie On School Food: 'I Don't Care' What Kids Eat," *The*

*Lunch Tray*, January 19, 2016, http://www.thelunchtray.com/ chris-christies-school-lunch-pandering/.

14    *American parents do support policies that…improve kids' health* Jennifer L. Harris, Karen S. Haraghey, Yoon-Young Choi, and Frances Fleming-Milici, "Parents' Attitudes About Food Marketing to Children: 2012 to 2015: Opportunities and Challenges to Creating Demand for a Healthier Food Environment," report from the UConn Rudd Center for Food Policy & Obesity, April 2017, http://www.uconnruddcenter.org/files/Pdfs/Rudd%20 Center%20Parent%20Attitudes%20Report%202017.pdf; "Parents Support Healthier School Food Policies by 3-to-1 Margin," Pew Charitable Trusts, Robert Wood Johnson Foundation, and American Heart Association, September 8, 2014, https://www.pewtrusts.org/en/about/news-room/press -releases-and-statements/2014/09/08/parents-support-healthier -school-food-policies-by-3to1-margin.

## 1. Kid Food: How Did We Get Here?

16    *online menu archives* The online menu archives I consulted are found at: the New York Public Library, http://menus.nypl.org/; the Los Angeles Public Library, https://www.lapl.org/ collections-resources/visual-collections/menu-collection; the Nestlé Library at Cornell University, https://sha.cornell.edu/ about/facilities/nestle-library/menus/; the Seattle Public Library, http://cdm16118.contentdm.oclc.org/cdm/landingpage/ collection/p16118coll5; the University of Washington's library, http://content.lib.washington.edu/menusweb/index.html; and the Culinary Institute of America, http://ciadigitalcollections .culinary.edu/digital/collection/p16940coll1. I also periodically searched eBay, where vintage children's menus are often available for purchase.

16    *paper on the role of children in the American restaurant industry* Andrew P. Haley, "Dining in High Chairs: Children and the American Restaurant Industry, 1900–1950," *Food and History* 7, no. 2 (2009): 69–94.

16 *"Why not children's luncheon?"* Ethel Colson, "Why Not Children's Luncheon?" *American Restaurant* 2, no. 3 (March 1920): 21.

16 *it "has never been done anywhere"* C. A. Patterson, "A Saturday Suggestion," *American Restaurant* 2, no. 3 (March 1920): 21.

16 *Colson ... was a writer* Illinois Women's Press Association, "The Lively Optimist," http://www.iwpa.org/the-lively-optimist/.

17 *teaching journalism to young women* "The Lively Optimist."

17 *"women's interests, ways and work"* Ethel C. Brazelton, *Writing and Editing for Women: A Bird's-Eye View of the Widening Opportunities for Women in Newspaper, Magazine and Other Writing Work* (New York: Funk & Wagnalls, 1927), 8.

17 *expert guidance on how to feed one's family* Susan Levine, *School Lunch Politics: The Surprising History of America's Favorite Social Welfare Program* (Princeton, NJ: Princeton University Press, 2008), 10–38; Helen Zoe Veit, "The Evolution of the American Diet," *Mother Earth News*, June 2014, https://www.motherearthnews.com/real-food/food-policy/american-diet-ze0z1406zcalt.

17 *"the growing child, the citizen of the future"* Colson, "Children's Luncheon," 21.

18 *Children were now occupying a more central role in family life* Haley, "Dining in High Chairs," 74.

18 *special meals for children* Haley, "Dining in High Chairs"; Jan Whitaker, "Children's Menus," *Restaurant-ing Through History*, April 22, 2018, https://restaurantingthroughhistory.com/2018/04/22/childrens-menus/.

18 *"tyrants" in "short jackets and pinafores"* Haley, "Dining in High Chairs," 71 (quoting "Undisciplined Children," *Chef* 8, no.12 [1898]: 564).

18 *refused to give parents any kind of price break* Haley, "Dining in High Chairs," 71–72.

18 *competition for diners was growing fierce* Haley, "Dining in High Chairs," 80–83.

19 *"will soon prove the financial feasibility of the idea"* "Little Children Lead them to Alice Foote MacDougall's," *Restaurant Man* 3, no. 3 (March 1928): 12.

19    *milk was considered the "best and most important food" for kids*
      Department of the Interior, Bureau of Education, *Diet for the
      School Child*, Health Education Series, No. 2 (Washington, DC:
      Government Printing Office, 1919), 3 (accessed through the
      Child Nutrition Archives, Institute of Child Nutrition, School
      of Applied Sciences at the University of Mississippi, http://
      archives.theicn.org/online-exhibitions/diet-for-the-school-
      child-health-education-no-2/).

19    *"the greaseless diet so beneficial to children"* William F. Donald,
      "They Find Profit in Catering to Kiddies," *Restaurant Man* 5, no.
      10 (October 1930): 22.

19    *she suggested serving "daintily cooked cereals..."* Colson,
      "Children's Luncheon," 21.

19    *"vegetable plate" or "vegetable luncheon"* I learned the meaning
      of these menu terms by consulting cookbooks from the same
      era. See, e.g., Wisconsin Farmers' Institutes, *A Hand-Book of
      Agriculture*, Bulletin No. 28 (1914), 312–20 ("Serving a Four-
      Course Vegetable Luncheon"); Ruth Berolzheimer, *The
      American Woman's Cook Book* (Chicago: Consolidated Book
      Publishers, Inc., 1939); General Electric Kitchen Institute, *The
      New Art of Modern Cooking* (1937), 17.

20    *when made to resemble an eyeball* Robert Clark, "Winning the
      Juvenile Patrons: Marshall Fields Profits by Catering to Tots,"
      *Restaurant Man* 4, no. 6 (June 1929): 13. Footnote: Maryn
      McKenna, "The Man Who Invented Chicken Nuggets—18
      Years Before McDonald's Did," *Slate*, December 28, 2012,
      http://www.slate.com/articles/life/food/2012/12/robert_c_
      baker_the_man_who_invented_chicken_nuggets.html.

20    *"vegetables that youngsters do not especially relish"* Clark,
      "Winning the Juvenile Patrons," 13.

20    *"Many of the [children's] dishes are selected for variety of color as
      well as flavor"* Donald, "Catering to Kiddies," 21.

21    *children's menu at Chili's ... Red Robin ... Friendly's* Information
      regarding these children's menus was found on the restaurants'
      respective websites.

21    *"good money" in feeding kids* Colson, "Children's Luncheon," 21.

21   *"especially attentive to Johnny"* Donald, "Catering to Kiddies," 21.

21   *non-food treats to lure kids in* Donald, "Catering to Kiddies," 21.

21   *decline in home cooking* United States Department of Agriculture, Economic Research Service, "U.S. Food-Away-From-Home Spending Continued to Outpace At-Home Spending in 2017," https://www.ers.usda.gov/data-products/chart-gallery/gallery/chart-detail/?chartId=58364; Matt Phillips, "No One Cooks Anymore," *Quartz*, June 14, 2016, https://qz.com/706550/no-one-cooks-anymore/?utm_source=nextdraft&utm_medium=email.

22   *"gum, squish, and swallow"* Melanie Potock, "Three Reasons Why Kids Get Hooked on 'Kids' Meals'...and How to Change That," *Leader Live—Happening Now in the Speech-Language-Hearing World*, July 3, 2014, blog.asha.org/2014/07/03/three-reasons-why-kids-get-hooked-on-kids-meals-and-how-to-change-that/.

23   *when breakfast cereal manufacturers started putting cartoon mascots* Heather Arndt Anderson, *Breakfast: A History* (Lanham, MD: AltaMira Press, 2013), 23.

23   *it wasn't until the mid-1990s to the early 2000s that "kid" versions of other kinds of foods* Michael J. McGinnis, *Food Marketing to Children and Youth: Threat or Opportunity?* (Washington, DC: National Academies Press, 2006) 156–62.

23   *breakfast cereal has lost its footing as the dominant "kid food" grocery category* Charlene D. Elliott, "Packaging Fun: Analyzing Supermarket Food Messages Targeted at Children," *Canadian Journal of Communication* 37, no. 2 (2012):303–18, doi:10.22230/cjc.2012v37n2a2550; market research commissioned by the author in 2018 from GlobalData, PLC, owner of the Products Launch Analytics database.

23   *since 2013, seven of the top eight product categories were sugary* Market research commissioned by the author in 2018 from GlobalData, PLC, owner of the Products Launch Analytics database.

23   *"kid food" products typically convey to children that they're in some way a form of entertainment* Elliott, "Packaging Fun."

23   *When children were asked in a 2012 focus group study*
Charlene D. Elliott, "'It's Junk Food and Chicken Nuggets':
Children's Perspectives on 'Kids' Food' and the Question of
Food Classification," *Journal of Consumer Behaviour* 10, no. 3
(2011): 133–40, doi:10.1002/cb.360.

24   *half of all American households with children reportedly buy
Goldfish* Andrew F. Smith, *Fast Food and Junk Food: An Encyclopedia
of What We Love to Eat* (Westport, CT: Greenwood, 2012), 311.

24   *foods like kidneys, lettuce, barley, and bone marrow* Clara Davis,
"Self-Selection of Diet By Newly Weaned Infants," *American
Journal of Diseases of Children* 36, no. 4 (October 1928): 651–78.

25   *put their kids on strict dietary regimens* See, e.g., L. Emmett
Holt, *The Care and Feeding of Children: A Catechism for the Use
of Mothers and Children's Nurses* (Toronto: McClelland &
Goodchild, 1907); Alan Gowans Brown, *The Normal Child; Its
Care and Feeding* (Toronto: McClelland and Stewart, 1932).

25   *50 to 90 percent of all pediatrician visits related to "anorexia"*
Stephen Strauss, "Clara M. Davis and the Wisdom of Letting
Children Choose Their Own Diets," *Canadian Medical
Association Journal* 175, no. 10 (July 2006): 1199–201.

25   *"theories, tastes or habits with respect to food"* Davis, "Self-
Selection of Diet By Newly Weaned Infants," 651–78.

26   *They were also told not to "comment on what he took..."* Ibid., 660.

26   *"until astonishingly large amounts were taken ... "* Ibid., 670.

26   *"the finest group of specimens...I have ever seen"* Clara Davis,
"Results of the Self-Selection of Diets By Young Children,"
*Canadian Medical Association Journal* 41 (September 1939):
257–61, at 259 (read at the 70th annual meeting of the Canadian
Medical Association, Section of Pediatrics, Montreal, June 21,
1939). Interestingly, in 1929, the *New York Times* reported on a
similar study conducted at Columbia University Teachers
College. The researchers in that (apparently unpublished) study
suspected that children would accept initially "distasteful" foods
if they were offered in an unemotional way, without bribery or
any discussion of the food's nutritional benefits. For four
months, children ranging in age from eighteen months through

three years were regularly offered tastes of liquids that were either pleasant, like chocolate, or unpleasant, like vinegar, and the liquids were offered "without conversation or exhortation." According to the *Times*, "At the end of the period the children took everything with apparent ease and indifference and seemed to have no particular aversion to any of the stimuli." "Told to Feed Child Without Emotions: Parents Advised in Survey Pleas and Promises Linked to Spinach Are Valueless," *New York Times*, June 3, 1929.

26    *"the altar of nutritional dogmatism"* Leo Kanner, *In Defense of Mothers; How to Bring up Children in Spite of the More Zealous Psychologists* (Springfield, IL: C. C. Thomas, 1941), 87–89.

27    *"can trust an unspoiled child's appetite"* Benjamin Spock, *The Common Sense Book of Baby and Child Care* (New York: Duell, Sloan and Pearce, 1945), 216–18.

27    *"novelty, cheapness, ease of procurement and preparation?"* Davis, "Results of the Self-Selection of Diets By Young Children," 261.

28    not *"just one token healthy option"* "Remarks by the First Lady in Address to the National Restaurant Association Meeting," National Archives and Records Administration, September 13, 2010, https://obamawhitehouse.archives.gov/the-press-office/2010/09/13/remarks-first-lady-address-national-restaurant-association-meeting.

28    *"healthful options for children"* Kids LiveWell website: https://www.restaurant.org/Industry-Impact/Food-Healthy-Living/Kids-LiveWell-Program.

28    *Kids LiveWell* Kids LiveWell program criteria accessed at: http://www.restaurant.org/Industry-Impact/Food-Healthy-Living/Kids-LiveWell/About.

28    *Silver Diner...embraced the challenge* Stephanie Anzman-Frasca et al., "Changes in Children's Meal Orders following Healthy Menu Modifications at a Regional US Restaurant Chain," *Obesity* 23, no. 5 (2015): 1055–62, doi:10.1002/oby.21061.

28    *several major restaurant chains have also recently dropped sugary drinks* Sara Ribakove, Jessica Almy, and Margo G. Wootan,

"Soda on the Menu: Improvements Seen But More Change Needed For Beverages On Restaurant Children's Menus," Center for Science in the Public Interest, July 2017, https://cspinet.org/kidsbeveragestudy.

29   *they still described their children's menus as "dismal" and basically unchanged* Alyssa Moran and Christina Roberto, "Restaurants Pledged to Make Kids' Meals Healthier—but the Data Show Not Much Has Changed," *Conversation*, May 29, 2018, https://theconversation.com/restaurants-pledged-to-make-kids-meals-healthier-but-the-data-show-not-much-has-changed-71761 (citing Alyssa J. Moran et al., "Trends in Nutrient Content of Children's Menu Items in U.S. Chain Restaurants," *American Journal of Preventive Medicine* 52, no. 3 [2017]: 284–91, doi:10.1016/j.amepre.2016.11.007).

29   *a 2017 study found...* Jennifer Harris et al., "Are Fast-Food Restaurants Keeping Their Promises to Offer Healthier Kids' Meals?" UConn Rudd Center for Food Policy & Obesity, August 2017, http://www.uconnruddcenter.org/files/Pdfs/272-9%20_%20Rudd_Healthier%20Kids%20Meals%20Report_Final%20Round_Web-150dpi_080117.pdf.

## 2. The Beige and the Bland

33   *there isn't a single supermarket nearby* Richard Florida, "Food Deserts Exist. But Do They Matter?" *Atlantic*, January 22, 2018, https://www.theatlantic.com/business/archive/2018/01/food-deserts/551138/ (citing Hunt Allcott, Rebecca Diamond, and Jean-Pierre Dubé, "The Geography of Poverty and Nutrition: Food Deserts and Food Choices Across the United States," National Bureau of Economic Research, Working Paper No. 24094 [December 2017], http://www.nber.org/papers/w24094).

33   *When families have to travel farther to shop* Sarah Bowen, Sinikka Elliott, and Joslyn Brenton, "The Joy of Cooking?" *Contexts* 13, no. 3 (2014): 20–25, doi:10.1177/1536504214545755.

33  *many parents don't have access to a car* Food Research and Action Center, "Understanding the Connections: Food Insecurity and Obesity," October 2015, http://frac.org/wp-content/uploads/frac_brief_understanding_the_connections.pdf (citing U.S. Department of Agriculture, Economic Research Service, "Access to Affordable and Nutritious Food: Measuring and Understanding Food Deserts and Their Consequences— Report to Congress").

34  *Other plant-eating animals...also experience food neophobia* Colin Barras, "It's Not Just Human Toddlers That Are Fussy Eaters," *BBC Earth*, April 3, 2017, http://www.bbc.com/earth/story/20170331-its-not-just-human-toddlers-that-are-fussy-eaters.

35  *This is especially true if they are prone to anxiety and shyness* Amy T. Galloway, Yoonna Lee, and Lean L. Birch, "Predictors and Consequences of Food Neophobia and Pickiness in Young Girls," *Journal of the American Dietetic Association* 103, no. 6 (2003): 692–98, doi:10.1053/jada.2003.50134; Andrea D. Smith et al., "Food Fussiness and Food Neophobia Share a Common Etiology in Early Childhood," *Journal of Child Psychology and Psychiatry* 58, no. 2 (2016): 189–96, doi:10.1111/jcpp.12647.

35  *The genetic link for selective eating* Alison Fildes et al., "Nature and Nurture in Children's Food Preferences," *American Journal of Clinical Nutrition* 99, no. 4 (2014): 911–17, doi:10.3945/ajcn.113.077867.

35  *just as adults are hardwired to seek out calorie-dense foods* Michael Moss, *Salt, Sugar, Fat: How the Food Giants Hooked Us* (New York: Random House, 2013); David A. Kessler, *The End of Overeating: Taking Control of the Insatiable American Appetite* (Waterville, ME: Thorndike Press, 2009).

35  *kids' tolerance for super-sweetness tends to peak during periods of rapid growth* Alison K. Ventura and Julie A. Mennella, "Innate and Learned Preferences for Sweet Taste During Childhood," *Current Opinion in Clinical Nutrition and Metabolic Care* 14, no. 4 (2011): 379–84, doi:10.1097/mco.0b013e328346df65;

Susan E. Coldwell, Teresa K. Oswald, and Danielle R. Reed, "A Marker of Growth Differs Between Adolescents with High vs. Low Sugar Preference," *Physiology & Behavior* 96, no. 4–5 (2009): 574–80, doi:10.1016/j.physbeh.2008.12.010.

36    *Sugar also has a pain-relieving effect in children* See the various studies cited in Julie A. Mennella and Nuala K. Bobowski, "The Sweetness and Bitterness of Childhood: Insights from Basic Research on Taste Preferences," *Physiology & Behavior* 152 (2015): 502–07, doi:10.1016/j.physbeh.2015.05.015.

36    *more likely even at age four to prefer savory snacks over sweet* Leslie J. Stein, Beverly J. Cowart, and Gary K. Beauchamp, "Development of Salty Taste Acceptance Is Related to Dietary Experience in Human Infants: A Prospective Study," *American Journal of Clinical Nutrition* 95, no. 1 (January 1, 2012): 123–29, doi:10.3945/ajcn.111.014282. A baby's in utero environment can also have this effect: if a mother suffers severe morning sickness during pregnancy, which is dehydrating, her child is more likely to be a salt-lover in adulthood, and the same is true for babies born with a low birth weight. See Susan R. Crystal and Ilene L. Bernstein, "Infant Salt Preference and Mothers' Morning Sickness," *Appetite* 30, no. 3 (1998): 297–307, doi:10.1006/appe.1997.0144; Leslie J. Stein, Beverly J. Cowart, Gary K. Beauchamp, "Salty Taste Acceptance by Infants and Young Children Is Related to Birth Weight: Longitudinal Analysis of Infants within the Normal Birth Weight Range," *European Journal of Clinical Nutrition* 60, no. 2 (2005): 272–79, doi:10.1038/sj.ejcn.1602312. See also Daniel Schwartz, "Why Toddler Foods Are Loaded with Sugar and Salt," *CBC News*, February 7, 2015, www.cbc.ca/news/health/why-toddler-foods-have-so-much-sugar-and-salt-1.2945353.

36    *researchers from the University of Tennessee* Betty Ruth Carruth, Paula J. Ziegler, Anne Gordon, and Susan I. Barr, "Prevalence of Picky Eaters among Infants and Toddlers and Their Caregivers' Decisions about Offering a New Food," *Journal of the American Dietetic Association* 104 (2004): 57–64, doi:10.1016/j.jada.2003.10.024.

36  *the study mentioned above found that many parents give up on offering a new food* Ibid.

36  *a poll of two thousand British parents found* "British Parents Are 'Giving Up' on Getting Kids to Eat Fruit and Vegetables, Survey Finds." *Independent*, May 10, 2018, www.independent.co.uk/ life-style/food-and-drink/news/healthy-eating-children-fruit-vegetables-five-a-day-families-nutrition-diet-a8344601.html (citing a survey conducted by the British appliance manufacturer Beko UK.)

37  *lower-income kids may get fewer opportunities* Caitlin Daniel, "Economic Constraints on Taste Formation and the True Cost of Healthy Eating," *Social Science & Medicine* 148 (January 2016): 34–41, doi:10.1016/j.socscimed.2015.11.025. See also Bowen, "The Joy of Cooking?" (Interviews with 150 mothers found that low-income women often stuck to cooking the same, less healthy foods rather than risk food waste.)

37  *According to the researchers, more affluent parents...* Priya Fielding-Singh, "A Taste of Inequality: Food's Symbolic Value across the Socioeconomic Spectrum," *Sociological Science* 4 (August 10, 2017): 424–48, doi:10.15195/v4.a17.

38  *kids in the pressured group were overwhelmingly negative* Amy T. Galloway, Laura M. Fiorito, Lori A. Francis, and Leann L. Birch, "'Finish Your Soup': Counterproductive Effects of Pressuring Children to Eat on Intake and Affect," *Appetite* 46, no. 3 (2006): 318–23, doi:10.1016/j.appet.2006.01.019.

38  *just telling a child how nutritious a food is...* "Avoid Pressure," Ellyn Satter Institute, https://www.ellynsatterinstitute.org/ how-to-feed/childhood-feeding-problems/#avoid-pressure.

38  *That's even more likely when a parent is herself a selective eater* Kameron J. Moding and Cynthia A. Stifter, "Stability of Food Neophobia from Infancy through Early Childhood," *Appetite* 97 (2016): 72–78, doi:10.1016/j.appet.2015.11.016.

39  *more recent research indicates that...an earlier introduction of peanuts is more effective* The American Academy of Allergy, Asthma & Immunology, "Newly Issued Clinical Guidelines from the NIAID Recommend Early Peanut Introduction, Not

Avoidance," January 5, 2017, www.aaaai.org/about-aaaai/
newsroom/news-releases/early-peanut-introduction. Babies are
considered high-risk if they have severe eczema, an egg allergy,
or both. Parents should of course seek medical advice before
following this new protocol.

39    *"the taproot of childhood obesity"* "White Out FAQ," *Dr. Greene,*
https://www.drgreene.com/whiteout-faq/#goal; for more on
the White Out Movement, see Amy Bentley, *Inventing Baby
Food: Taste, Health, and the Industrialization of the American Diet*
(Oakland: University of California Press, 2014), 158–59.

39    *Rice cereal may also contain excessive amounts of naturally
occurring arsenic* Roni Caryn Rabin, "Should You Be Worried
About the Arsenic in Your Baby Food?" *New York Times,*
December 7, 2017, https://www.nytimes.com/2017/12/07/
well/eat/should-you-be-worried-about-the-arsenic-in-your-baby-
food.html; Trisha Korioth, "Parent Plus: Limit Infants' Exposure
to Arsenic By Feeding a Variety of Grains," *AAP News,* May 19,
2016, https://www.aappublications.org/news/2016/05/19/
Arsenic051916.

39    *the optimal period for accepting new flavors is between four
and six months* Helen Coulthard, Gillian Harris, and Anna
Fogel, "Exposure to Vegetable Variety in Infants Weaned at
Different Ages," *Appetite* 78 (2014): 89–94, doi:10.1016/j.
appet.2014.03.021; Alison Fildes et al., "An Exploratory Trial
of Parental Advice for Increasing Vegetable Acceptance in
Infancy," *British Journal of Nutrition* 114, no. 2 (2015): 328–36,
doi:10.1017/s0007114515001695.

39    *willingness to accept new flavors . . . increases when they're
exposed to a wider variety of new tastes* Andrea Maier-Nöth,
Benoist Schaal, Peter Leathwood, and Sylvie Issanchou, "The
Lasting Influences of Early Food-Related Variety Experience:
A Longitudinal Study of Vegetable Acceptance from 5 Months
to 6 Years in Two Populations," *PLOS ONE* 11, no. 3 (2016),
doi:10.1371/journal.pone.0151356.

40    *In one study, when moms frequently drank carrot juice* Gretchen
Cuda-Kroen, "Baby's Palate and Food Memories Shaped Before

Birth," *NPR*, August 8, 2011, https://www.npr.org/2011/08/08/ 139033757/babys-palate-and-food-memories-shaped-before-birth; Julie A. Mennella, Coren P. Jagnow, and Gary K. Beauchamp, "Prenatal and Postnatal Flavor Learning by Human Infants," *Pediatrics* 107, no. 6 (2001), doi:10.1542/peds.107.6.e88.

40    *one study found that if a pregnant rat was fed*... Z. Y. Ong and B. S. Muhlhausler, "Maternal 'Junk-Food' Feeding of Rat Dams Alters Food Choices and Development of the Mesolimbic Reward Pathway in the Offspring," *FASEB Journal* 25, no. 7 (2011): 2167–79, doi:10.1096/fj.10-178392.

41    *in that same carrot juice study* Mennella, Jagnow, and Beauchamp, "Prenatal and Postnatal Flavor Learning by Human Infants."

41    *formula-fed babies are less likely to embrace new tastes* Julie A. Mennella and Sara M. Castor, "Sensitive Period in Flavor Learning: Effects of Duration of Exposure to Formula Flavors on Food Likes During Infancy," *Clinical Nutrition* 31, no. 6 (December 2012): 1022–25, doi:10.1016/j.clnu.2012.05.005.

41    *the "flavor window" from Bee Wilson's excellent book* Bee Wilson, *First Bite: How We Learn to Eat* (New York: Basic Books, 2016).

42    *"Division of Responsibility" (DOR)* Ellyn Satter, *Child of Mine: Feeding with Love and Good Sense* (Boulder, CO: Bull Publishing, 2000).

42    *"She is growing up to join you at your family table"* Satter, *Child of Mine*, 12.

42    *preschoolers were more likely to eat a colored porridge with an unfamiliar flavor* Elsa Addessi, Amy T. Galloway, Elisabetta Visalberghi, and Leann L. Birch, "Specific Social Influences on the Acceptance of Novel Foods in 2- to 5-year-old Children," *Appetite* 45, no. 3 (2005): 264–71, doi:10.1016/j.appet.2005.07.007.

42    *70 percent of moms now work outside the home* U.S. Department of Labor, Bureau of Labor Statistics, news release, April 19, 2018, https://www.bls.gov/news.release/pdf/famee.pdf.

43    *according to one study of millennial mothers* Christine Michel Carter, "Meet The Company Decoding How to Market to Millennial Moms," *Forbes*, February 1, 2018, https://www .forbes.com/sites/christinecarter/2017/05/01/marketing-to-

millennial-moms-where-there-is-pain-there-is-profit
/#704537bf5201.

43   *a recent Pew report found* Pew Research Center, "Parenting in America: Outlook, Worries, Aspirations Are Strongly Linked to Financial Situation," December 17, 2015, http://www .pewsocialtrends.org/2015/12/17/parenting-in-america/.

43   *one out of five meals eaten by kids* Carter, "Millennial Moms."

44   *when a meal was prepared mainly with fresh ingredients* Elinor Ochs and Tamar Kremer-Sadlik, *Fast-Forward Family: Home, Work, and Relationships in Middle-Class America* (Berkeley: University of California Press, 2013), 48–65.

44   *CELF researches also noted* Ochs and Kremer-Sadlik, *Fast-Forward Family*, 64.

44   *almost one-third of all baby food is eaten from a pouch* Bentley, *Inventing Baby Food*, 149–51; Matt Richtel, "Food Pouches Let Little Ones Serve Themselves," *New York Times*, June 20, 2012, https://www.nytimes.com/2012/06/21/garden/food-pouches-let-little-ones-serve-themselves.html.

44   *lack of structure around eating can quickly undermine the DOR* Richtel, "Food Pouches"; Melinda Wenner Moyer, "Puréed Fruit Pouches Are Not God's Gift to Children's Snacks," *Slate*, March 27, 2013, www.slate.com/articles/double_x/the_kids/2013/03/pure_organic_buddyfruit_the_case_against_blended_fruit_snacks.html.

45   *guidance on handling picky eating from a 1825 parenting treatise* William P. Dewees, *A Treatise on the Physical and Medical Treatment of Children* (Philadelphia: H .C. Carey and I. Lea, 1825), 205.

46   *parent-child exchange about dinner, documented by the CELF researchers* Ochs and Kremer-Sadlik, *Fast-Forward Family*, 54.

46   *kids' taste preferences influenced 95 percent of parents food and beverage purchase decisions* Carolyn Heneghan, "Children's Picky Palates Drive Parents' Grocery Purchases," *Food Dive*, August 3, 2016, https://www.fooddive.com/news/childrens-picky-palates-drive-parents-grocery-purchases/423759/.

46   *"You know more about the food in the world than she does"* Satter, *Child of Mine*, 12.

# 3. The Claim Game

51     *Tyson is hardly the only company using this approach* Tyson "Trying Everything" commercial accessed at https://www.ispot. tv/ad/7K7W/tyson-crispy-chicken-strips-trying-everything; Tyson "Picky Eaters" chicken nugget commercial accessed at https://www.ispot.tv/ad/75Jf/tyson-fun-nuggets-picky-eaters; Tyson "I Hate Everything" commercial accessed at https:// www.youtube.com/watch?v=nM8oyrKY_ZE; Eggo waffles commercial accessed at https://www.youtube.com/watch?v =e2A8SrvjMKE; Ore-Ida commercial accessed at https:// www.youtube.com/watch?v=x8ZUvU_SW-I&feature =youtube. (Ore-Ida even offered parents a Potato Pay "currency" chart: http://www.trypotatopay.com/.)

51     *Kid Cuisine . . . a KFC ad* Kid Cuisine website, www.kidcuisine. com; Bettina Elias Siegel, "Kraft Ads Tell Parents: Just Give Up, Kids Won't Eat Healthier Foods," *The Lunch Tray*, April 30, 2019, https://www.thelunchtray.com/kraft-ads-tell-parents-just-give-up-kids-wont-eat-healthier-food/; "Abbott's PediaSure® Brand Aims to Help Moms With Picky Eaters 'Take Back the Table' By Building Lifelong Healthy Eating Habits," *FiercePharma*, August 11, 2011, https://www.fiercepharma.com/pharma/abbott-s-pediasure®-brand-aims-to-help-moms-picky-eaters-take-back-table-by-building; KFC ad, "Dipping Is Fun," accessed at https:// www.ispot.tv/ad/7SOn/kfc-dipems-bucket-dipping-is-fun.

52     *Kraft Heinz . . . a sugary snack bar* Siegel, "Kraft Ads Tell Parents: Just Give Up"; Chef Boyardee ad campaign accessed at https://www.adsoftheworld.com/campaign/chef-boyardee-ddb-09-2010; promotional copy for Similac Go and Grow, accessed at https://abbottstore.com/go-grow-similac-milk-based-powder-toddler-drink-2lb-case-of-6-66386.html; Healthbar Kids promotional video accessed at https://www.youtube.com/ watch?v=uT7gHvwblV8.

52     *A recent focus group study found* Katie M. Abrams, Caitlin Evans, and Brittany R. L. Duff, "Ignorance Is Bliss: How Parents of Preschool Children Make Sense of Front-of-Package Visuals

and Claims on Food," *Appetite* 87, no. 1 (April 1, 2015): 20–29, doi:10.1016/j.appet.2014.12.100.

53 *"gluten free"* In 2014, late night host Jimmy Kimmel asked random passers-by in Los Angeles to define "gluten" and explain why they avoid it. Many appeared to be confused, to say the least. https://www.youtube.com/watch?v=AdJFE1sp4Fw.

53 *nutritional criteria set by the Food and Drug Administration* As of this writing, the Food and Drug Administration is seeking public comment on redefining the nutritional criteria for making a "healthy" claim. Right now, some healthy foods like salmon and nuts don't qualify due to their fat content, while a highly processed food like fat-free pudding could qualify.

53 *A recent study of baby and toddler foods* UConn Rudd Center for Food Policy & Obesity, "Baby Food FACTS: Nutrition and Marketing of Baby and Toddler Food and Drinks," January 2017, accessed at http://www.uconnruddcenter.org/files/Pdfs/BabyFoodFACTS_FINAL.pdf.

53 *"If you're concerned about your health, you should probably avoid products that make health claims"* Michael Pollan, *In Defense of Food: An Eater's Manifesto* (New York: Penguin Press, 2009), 12.

54 *A Nielsen study broke it down even further* Nielsen, "Back to School for Students, and Back to the Grocery Aisles for Parents," August 15, 2016, https://www.nielsen.com/us/en/insights/news/2016/back-to-school-and-back-to-the-grocery-aisles.html.

54 *Nutrient claims like these are legal... Welch's blueberry Fruit'n Yogurt snacks* Center for Science in the Public Interest, "Phony Fruit Snacks," https://cspinet.org/phony-fruit-snacks; Welch's Fruit'n Yogurt snacks ingredient listing found at https://www.welchsfruitsnacks.com/products/blueberry-yogurt/.

54 *at least one study indicates* Prevention Institute, "Claiming Health: Front-of-Package Labeling of Children's Food," January 1, 2011, http://www.preventioninstitute.org/publications/claiming-health-front-of-package-labeling-of-childrens-food.

55 *Girl Scouts' Mango Creme sandwich cookie* Bettina Elias Siegel, "A Girl Scout Cookie Gets 'Healthwashed,' And Some Musings on Nutritionism and Our Kids," *The Lunch Tray*, January 17, 2013.

55    *The marketing ploy was widely criticized* Center for Science in the Public Interest, "CSPI Letter to Girl Scouts of the USA Re: Misleading Labeling," February 8, 2013, https://cspinet. org/resource/cspi-letter-girl-scouts-usa-re-misleading-labeling; Caity Weaver, "The New Girl Scout Cookie Tastes Like BULLSHIT," *Gawker*, January 11, 2013, http://gawker. com/5975288/the-new-girl-scout-cookie-tastes-like-bullshit.

55    *Veggie Booty... "Good for You"* Original Veggie Booty package copy found at http://www.taquitos.net/snacks.php?snack_code=584.

55    *"baby crack"* Mary Elizabeth Williams, "Bootylicious," *Salon*, September 25, 2011, https://www.salon.com/2005/06/08/object_lust4/. Footnote: Rob Walker, "Snack Mentality," *New York Times*, June 28, 2008, http://www.nytimes.com/2008/06/29/magazine/29wwln-consumed-t.html.

56    *Gerber... Organic Farm Greens Veggie Crisps* Nutritional information for Gerber Veggie Crisps found at https://thegerberstore.com/organic-veggie-crisps-farm-greens/GER+00015000120023.html?trk_src_ss=GERPAYPCWEB MACSS&gclid=CjwKCAjwkMbaBRBAEiwAlH5v_hfeee2PQTXkhk-V1SXMULJQ_08lPJt_tcoNjXZ-ZQpYlhTY4pwPuhoCKQAQAvD_BwE.

56    *Plum Organics's Super Puffs with Blueberry and Purple Sweet Potato* Nutrition information for Plum Organics Super Puffs found at https://www.plumorganics.com/products/super-purples-blueberry-purple-sweet-potato/.

56    *"because they can finally get their kids to eat vegetables"* Cara Rosenbloom, "Six Foods That Marketers Want You to Think Are Healthy," *Washington Post*, August 14, 2017, https://www.washingtonpost.com/lifestyle/wellness/how-many-of-these-6-foods-have-marketers-tricked-you-into-thinking-are-healthy/2017/08/11/87cfc832-70bd-11e7-9eac-d56bd5568db8_story.html?utm_term=.f08c11d7f8b1.

56    *Chef Boyardee campaign* Jennifer LaRue Huget, "Is That Right? Chef Boyardee Whole-Grain Beefaroni Is 'Secretly Nutritious,'"

*Washington Post*, August 27, 2010 (the author found that the products contained so much fat and sodium, they were still a bad nutritional deal for children).

56   *Kidfresh... The brand OH YES!* Bettina Elias Siegel, "Should the Food Industry Sneak Vegetables Into Food?" *New York Times*, October 25, 2016, https://www.nytimes.com/2016/10/25/well/eat/should-the-food-industry-sneak-vegetables-into-food.html; Ellen Shoup, "Kidfresh to Launch Organic Products and Debut Brand Refresh by End of Year," *Food Navigator USA*, June 22, 2018, https://www.foodnavigator-usa.com/Article/2018/06/22/Kidfresh-to-launch-organic-products-and-debut-brand-refresh-by-end-of-year.

57   *In 2015, the industry spent $9 million* Heather Timmons, "Breastfeeding Is Winning! So Companies Are Pushing 'Toddler Milk' to Neurotic Parents," *Quartz*, February 10, 2014, https://qz.com/171410/breastfeeding-is-winning-so-companies-are-pushing-toddler-milk-to-create-little-geniuses; UConn Rudd Center for Food Policy & Obesity, "Baby Food FACTS."

57   *As of 2014, toddler beverages were a $15 billion business* Timmons, "Breastfeeding Is Winning!"

57   *more than 40 percent of American parents offer toddler drinks* Timmons, "Breastfeeding Is Winning!"; Lauren Weber, "Toddler Formula Is Unnecessary. So Why Is It So Popular?" *Huffington Post*, August 11, 2018, https://www.huffingtonpost.com/entry/toddler-formula-milk-breastfeeding_us_5b69bd70e4b0fd5c73ddf505.

58   *experts say these... have no place in a child's healthy diet* Jennifer L. Pomeranz, Maria J. Romo Palafox, and Jennifer L. Harris, "Toddler Drinks, Formulas, and Milks: Labeling Practices and Policy Implications," *Preventative Medicine* 109 (April 2018): 11–16, doi:10.1016/j.ypmed.2018.01.009.

58   *all kinds of questionable claims* Promotional copy for Enfamil Premium Toddler Transitions, accessed at https://www.enfamil.com/products/enfagrow-premium-toddler-transitions; promotional copy for Enfagrow Premium Toddler Next Step

accessed at https://www.enfamil.com/products/enfagrow-premium-toddler-next-step-natural-milk/24-oz-powder-can-case-4?gclid=CjwKCAjwh9_bBRA_EiwApObaOKaGP_XfrZy2BZkLTGuRybz5M0Z83a-lydA-sQAYVB6JAb8p0l8mqBoCLagQAvD_BwE.

58    *"fill any nutritional gaps"* Promotional copy for Gerber Good Start Grow Nutritious toddler drink powder accessed at https://www.gerber.com/toddler/articles/say-hello-to-milk-juice/nutritional-assurance-for-toddlers.

59    *"to help balance out a picky eater's uneven diet"* "Abbott Launches Pediasure SideKicks Clear For Picky Eaters," May 16, 2012, http://abbott.mediaroom.com/2012-05-16-Abbott-Launches-PediaSure-SideKicks-Clear-for-Picky-Eaters"; Abbott's SideKicks web page: https://pediasure.com/nutrition-drinks-for-kids/sidekicks-nutrition-shakes.

59    *Abbott created a "PediaSure Mom Brigade"* "Abbott's PediaSure Brand Aims to Help Moms," *FiercePharma.*

59    *a commercial Abbott was forced to pull* "A.G. Schneiderman Announces Settlement with Maker of PediaSure SideKicks Supplement for Misleading Advertising," press release from the office of the New York State Attorney General, December 4, 2013, https://ag.ny.gov/press-release/ag-schneiderman-announces-settlement-maker-pediasure-sidekicks-supplement-misleading.

59    *"Good old-fashioned guilt"* Quote found at *The Book of Larry,* http://www.thebookoflarry.com/broadcastvideo.html.

60    *A key strategy…has been funding academic studies that "medicalize" children's picky eating* Veronica Sau-Wa Mak, "How Picky Eating Becomes an Illness—Marketing Nutrient-Enriched Formula Milk in a Chinese Society," *Ecology of Food and Nutrition* 56, no. 1 (February 2017): 81–100, doi:10.1080/03670244.2016.1261025.

60    *According to Mak, a 2003 survey found* Mak, "How Picky Eating Becomes an Illness," 87-88.

60    *"underestimated the impact of [picky eating] symptoms"* Jennifer Chan, "Leo Burnett Launches First Work for Abbott PediaSure,"

*Marketing Interactive*, December 18, 2013, https://www.marketing-interactive.com/leo-burnett-launches-first-campaign-new-account-abbott/. In other countries, Abbott makes even more aggressive health claims for PediaSure. In South Africa, for example, the company promotes it as a "solution" to "fussy or picky eating" but also implies that one PediaSure variant boosts immunity and significantly lessens the symptoms of cold and flu. See "Toddler Picky Eating," https://nutrition.abbott/za/continuing-education/child-nutrition/toddler-picky-eating.

60   *Another advertising industry article noted* Benjamin Li, "Abbott Strives to Smash Picky-Eating Myths," *Campaign Asia*, December 17, 2013, https://www.campaignasia.com/video/abbott-strives-to-smash-picky-eating-myths/367833.

61   *do eggs cause heart attacks or are they healthy now?* A 2017 Funny or Die video, in which a time-traveling dietitian offers a 1979 couple ever-changing dietary advice, says it all: http://www.funnyordie.com/videos/74dd9afee2/time-travel-dietician-this-is-why-eating-healthy-is-hard.

61   *apples and kale are healthy while soda and cookies aren't* Kevin Quealy and Margot Sanger-Katz, "Is Sushi 'Healthy'? What About Granola? Where Americans and Nutritionists Disagree," *New York Times*, July 5, 2016, https://www.nytimes.com/interactive/2016/07/05/upshot/is-sushi-healthy-what-about-granola-where-americans-and-nutritionists-disagree.html.

62   *the study was funded by the National Confectioners Association* Candice Choi, "AP Exclusive: How Candy Makers Shape Nutrition Science," *AP News*, June 2, 2016, https://apnews.com/f9483d554430445fa6566bb0aaa293d1.

62   *examples...funded by Quaker Oats...funded by Sabra...funded by Welch's* Candida J. Rebello et al., "Instant Oatmeal Increases Satiety and Reduces Energy Intake Compared to a Ready-to-Eat Oat-Based Breakfast Cereal: A Randomized Crossover Trial," *Journal of the American College of Nutrition* 35, no. 1 (2015): 41–49, doi:10.1080/07315724.2015.1032442; Carol E. O'Neil, Theresa A. Nicklas, and Victor L. Fulgoni III,

"Chickpeas and Hummus Are Associated with Better Nutrient Intake, Diet Quality, and Levels of Some Cardiovascular Risk Factors: National Health and Nutrition Examination Survey 2003–2010," *Journal of Nutrition & Food Sciences* 4, no. 1 (2014), doi:10.4172/2155-9600.1000254; Daniel J. Lamport et al., "Concord Grape Juice, Cognitive Function, and Driving Performance: a 12-Wk, Placebo-Controlled, Randomized Crossover Trial on Mothers of Preteen Children," *American Journal of Clinical Nutrition* 103, no. 3 (March 2016): 775–83, doi:10.3945/ajcn.115.114553.

62  *in 2018, researchers reviewed fifteen years' worth of studies* Dean Schillinger, Jessica Tran, Christina Mangurian, and Cristin Kearns, "Do Sugar-Sweetened Beverages Cause Obesity and Diabetes? Industry and the Manufacture of Scientific Controversy," *Annals of Internal Medicine* 165, no. 12 (2016): 895, doi:10.7326/l16-0534.

63  *a running score of all the industry-sponsored studies* Marion Nestle, "Food Industry Funding of Nutrition Research," *JAMA Internal Medicine* 176, no. 11 (2016): 1685, doi:10.1001/jamainternmed.2016.5400. Nestle has since written a book devoted to the topic of industry influence in nutrition research: Marion Nestle, *Unsavory Truth: How Food Companies Skew the Science of What We Eat* (New York: Basic Books, 2018). Another potential issue is a failure to disclose industry ties at all. See, e.g., Gary Ruskin, "Did 24 Coke-Funded Studies on Childhood Obesity Fail to Disclose Coke's Influence?" *U.S. Right to Know*, December 11, 2017, https://usrtk.org/news-releases/did-24-coke-funded-studies-on-childhood-obesity-fail-to-disclose-cokes-influence/.

63  *Coca-Cola also provided millions to the Global Energy Balance Network* Anahad O'Connor, "Coca-Cola Funds Scientists Who Shift Blame for Obesity Away From Bad Diets," *New York Times*, August 9, 2015, https://well.blogs.nytimes.com/2015/08/09/coca-cola-funds-scientists-who-shift-blame-for-obesity-away-from-bad-diets/; Anahad O'Connor, "Research Group Funded by Coca-Cola to Disband," *New York*

*Times*, December 1, 2015, https://well.blogs.nytimes.com/2015/12/01/research-group-funded-by-coca-cola-to-disband/.

63  *"junk science"* See, e.g., Rob A. Moodie, "What Public Health Practitioners Need to Know About Unhealthy Industry Tactics," *American Journal of Public Health* 107, no. 7 (2017): 1047–49, doi:10.2105/ajph.2017.303861; Kelly D. Brownell and Kenneth E. Warner, "The Perils of Ignoring History: Big Tobacco Played Dirty and Millions Died. How Similar Is Big Food?" *Milbank Quarterly* 87, no. 1 (2009): 259–94, doi:10.1111/j.1468-0009.2009.00555.x.

63  *no fewer than twenty paid experts to tell the media there was "conflicting science"* Deena Shanker, "Emails Show How the Food Industry Uses 'Science' to Push Soda," *Bloomberg*, September 13, 2017, https://www.bloomberg.com/news/articles/2017-09-13/emails-show-how-the-food-industry-uses-science-to-push-soda.

64  *millions of dollars being spent in these ways to keep us guessing about who's really telling the truth* Kari Hamerschlag, Anna Lappé, and Stacy Malkan, "Spinning Food: How Food Industry Front Groups and Covert Communications Are Shaping the Story of Food," *Friends of the Earth*, June 2015, https://foe.org/projects/food-and-technology/good-food-healthy-planet/spinning-food. ("The industrial food and agricultural sector spent hundreds of millions of dollars from 2009 to 2013 on communications efforts to spin the media, drive consumer behavior and advance its policy agenda. Spending includes $126 million spent by 14 food industry front groups that often appear in the media as independent sources but are funded by and serve the interests of the industrial food sector."); Michele Simon, "Best Public Relations Money Can Buy: A Guide to Food Industry Front Groups," *EatDrinkPolitics*, http://www.eatdrinkpolitics.com/reports/food-industry/examples-of-food-industry-front-groups/; Andy Kroll and Jeremy Schulman, "Leaked documents reveal the secret finances of a pro-industry science group," *Mother Jones*, July 12, 2017, http://www

.motherjones.com/politics/2013/10/american-council-science-health-leaked-documents-fundraising/.

64  *registered dietitian offering that nutritional advice just happens to be paid by Coca-Cola* Candice Choi, "Coca-Cola Paid Nutrition Experts to Recommend Soda as a Healthy Snack," *Business Insider*, March 16, 2015, http://www.businessinsider.com/coca-cola-paid-nutrition-experts-to-recommend-soda-as-a-healthy-snack-2015-3.

64  *the food and beverage industries...cozy up to the Academy of Nutrition and Dietetics* Michele Simon, "And Now a Word from Our Sponsors," *EatDrinkPolitics*, January 23, 2013, http://www.eatdrinkpolitics.com/2013/01/22/and-now-a-word-from-our-sponsors-new-report-from-eat-drink-politics/.

65  *"Mom bloggers" and popular mom Instagrammers are also aggressively courted* Christine Michel Carter, "Millennial Moms: The $2.4 Trillion Social Media Influencer," *Forbes*, October 17, 2017 https://www.forbes.com/sites/christinecarter/2017/06/15/millennial-moms-the-2-4-trillion-social-media-influencer/#2e8f27742261; Jennifer Calfas, "The New Mommy Blogger: Instagram Famous, Highly Paid, and Sponsored By Minute Maid," May 11, 2018, *Money*, http://money.com/money/5269576/mommy-bloggers-success/.

65  *glowing blog posts* Janine Huldie, "5 Reasons Why Your Family Needs to Visit McDonald's," June 7, 2017, https://www.janinehuldie.com/2017/06/5-reasons-family-visit-mcdonalds/; Karin Swanson, "McDonald's Influencer Strategy: We're Lovin' It!" *Medium*, February 6, 2017, https://medium.com/juliusworks/mcdonalds-influencer-strategy-we-re-lovin-it-7140213cd13b.

65  *nonetheless a paid-for post with a misleading "healthy" message* Sarah L. Lampley, "Snacking on the Go" (undated), https://www.sarahllampley.com/motherhood/snacking-on-the-go.

66  *Mom influencers are also sometimes co-opted by the industry on matters of scientific debate* Anna Lappé, "Big Food Uses Mommy Bloggers to Shape Public Opinion," *Al Jazeera America*, August 1, 2014, http://america.aljazeera.com/opinions/2014/8/food-

agriculturemonsantogmoadvertising.html; Melanie Warner, "High Fructose Corn Syrup's Latest PR Target: Mommy Bloggers," *CBS News*, October 15, 2010, http://www.cbsnews.com/news/high-fructose-corn-syrups-latest-pr-target-mommy-bloggers/.

68  *"sticking around to play branded games"* All of the quotes and information relayed here regarding the 2010 Kid Cuisine reboot accessed on the Geppetto Group website at https://www.geppettogroup.com/portfolio/kid-cuisine/; https://www.geppettogroup.com/portfolio/kid-cuisine-kc/; and https://www.geppettogroup.com/portfolio/kid-cuisine-digital/.

## 4. Pester Power

70  *Studies have also found that kids beg for a desired product an average of nine times* All supporting studies cited in K. M. Holly, Henry Borzekowski, and Dina L. G. Borzekowski, "The Nag Factor," *Journal of Children and Media* 5, no. 3 (2011): 298–317, doi:10.1080/17482798.2011.584380, with the exception of data regarding the types of foods kids request most often, which was found in: Michael J. McGinnis, *Food Marketing to Children and Youth: Threat or Opportunity?* (Washington, DC: National Academies Press, 2006) 102–3.

70  *the first-ever toy commercial, for Mr. Potato Head, ran on television* Jon Kelly, "Is Mr. Potato Head to Blame for 'Pester Power' Ads?" *BBC News*, April 30, 2012, www.bbc.com/news/magazine-17871107.

70  *according to social historian Lisa Jacobson* Lisa Jacobson, *Raising Consumers: Children and the American Mass Market in the Early Twentieth Century* (New York: Columbia University Press, 2004) 17–55.

70  *kids "have a way of…getting what they set their hearts on"* Jacobson, *Raising Consumers*, 16.

70  *"[W]ho can long resist the appeal of a child filled with great desire?"* Jacobson, *Raising Consumers*, 30–32.

71  *"because she's the nicest person in the world…except maybe you"* Jacobson, *Raising Consumers*, 46–50.

71    *ads should influence the parent-child relationship only "in a constructive manner"* "The Self-Regulatory Program for Children's Advertising," Children's Advertising Review Unit of the Council of Better Business Bureaus, accessed at http://www.caru.org/guidelines/index.aspx.

71    *an executive at the global ad agency, Saatchi & Saatchi* Mary Novakovich, "The Playground Pound," *Guardian*, November 3, 1999, www.theguardian.com/media/1999/nov/03/tvandradio.g2.

71    *a marketing executive speaking about a study called "The Nag Factor"* Erik Curren, "Meet the Woman Who Makes Your Kids Nag You for Products," *Transition Voice*, January 5, 2012, transitionvoice.com/2012/01/meet-the-woman-who-makes-your-kids-nag-you-for-products/(quoting an excerpt from the 2003 documentary film, *The Corporation*.)

71    *a senior brand manager at Heinz* Jonathan Eig, "Food Companies Grab Kids' Attention By Packaging Products as Toys, Games," *Wall Street Journal*, October 24, 2001, ww.wsj.com/articles/SB1003877010689858680.

72    *Children...spend around $40 billion a year, while teens spend almost $160 billion* Pester Power and children's spending data found at Campaign for a Commercial-Free Childhood, https://www.commercialfreechildhood.org/resource/marketing-children-overview.

72    *research shows that brand preferences formed in childhood tend to last a lifetime* Patti M. Valkenburg and Joanne Cantor, "The Development of a Child into a Consumer," *Journal of Applied Developmental Psychology* 22, no. 1 (2001): 61–72, doi:10.1016/s0193-3973(00)00066-6.

72    *before the age of six, because that's when "brand loyalty begins"* PR Newswire, "Packaged Facts: Kids Control Household Food Purchase Choices," August 8, 2016, http://www.prnewswire.com/news-releases/packaged-facts-kids-control-household-food-purchase-choices-300309936.html.

72    *had collectively spent $1.8 billion that year to market their brands just to children* Federal Trade Commission, "A Review of Food Marketing to Children and Adolescents:

Follow Up Report" (2012) ES-1, accessed at https://www.ftc. gov/sites/default/files/documents/reports/review-food-marketing-children-and-adolescents-follow-report/121221 foodmarketingreport.pdf.

72 *"...The food industry spends that amount [on child-directed marketing] by January 4th"* "Pounding Away at America's Obesity Epidemic," *Fresh Air*, NPR, May 14, 2012, https://www.npr.org/2012/05/14/152667325/pounding-away-at-americas-obesity-epidemic.

73 *a widely read 1997 book* Dan S. Acuff and Robert H. Reiher, *What Kids Buy and Why: The Psychology of Marketing to Kids* (New York: Free Press, 1997).

73 *advice on how to reach the "birth-to-two-year-old" set* Ibid., 168.

73 *"marketers were interested in using brain science and media psychology to sell more stuff"* Juliet Schor, *Born To Buy: The Commercialized Child and the New Consumer Culture* (New York: Scribner, 2004) 111–12.

73 *ad agency Saatchi & Saatchi once hired a team of clinical psychologists and cultural anthropologists* Susan Linn, "Sellouts," *American Prospect*, November 7, 2001, http://prospect.org/article/sellouts; Dale Russakoff, "For Marketers, Youth Trend Is No Child's Play," *Washington Post*, April 19, 1999.

74 *"establish limits...regarding the use of psychological knowledge or techniques to observe, study, etc."* Constance L. Hays, "A Call for Restrictions on Psychological Research by Advertisers into Products for Children," *New York Times*, October 22, 1999, www.nytimes.com/1999/10/22/business/media-business-advertising-call-for-restrictions-psychological-research.html. The text of the 1999 letter sent to the American Psychological Association is archived at Commercial Alert, "Psychologists, Psychiatrists Call for Limits on the Use of Psychology to Influence or Exploit Children for Commercial Purposes," archive.commercialalert.org/news/news-releases/1999/09/commercial-alert-psychologists-psychiatrists-call-for-limits-on-the-use-of-psychology-to-influence-or-exploit-children-for-commercial-purposes.

74 *will offer clients "new tools and pathways" to reach children* Next Step website, https://www.nextstepstrat.com.

74 *"translate genuine child development insights into business-growing ideas"* The Geppetto Group website, https://www.geppettogroup.com.

74 *once forged, this emotional connection "is basically impossible to get rid of"* Carina Storrs, "Kids Seeing More Unhealthy Snack Ads, Report Says," *CNN*, November 2, 2015, www.cnn.com/2015/11/02/health/children-snack-food-advertising/index.html.

74 *an effect that's unfortunately stronger for junk food* Matthew A. Lapierre et al., "Influence of Licensed Spokescharacters and Health Cues on Children's Ratings of Cereal Taste," *Archives of Pediatrics & Adolescent Medicine* 165, no. 3 (January 2011), doi:10.1001/archpediatrics.2010.300; Christina Roberto, Jenny Baik, Jennifer L. Harris, and Kelly D. Brownell, "Influence of Licensed Characters on Children's Taste and Snack Preferences," *Pediatrics* 126, no. 1 (2010): 88–93, doi:10.1542/peds.2009-3433.

75 *"I avoid ads, but she still notices, and [the ads] are manipulative"* Henry and Borzekowski, "The Nag Factor."

75 *"but the parents should do so only rarely"* Dan S. Acuff and Robert H. Reiher, *Kidnapped: How Irresponsible Marketers Are Stealing the Minds of Your Children* (Chicago: Dearborn Publishing Group, 2005), 109.

75 *a 2016 study looked at the products associated with kids' favorite music stars* Marie A. Bragg et al., "Popular Music Celebrity Endorsements in Food and Nonalcoholic Beverage Marketing," *Pediatrics* 138, no. 1 (June 2016), doi:10.1542/peds.2015-3977.

75 *star athletes...seem to have no qualms about promoting junk food* Marie A. Bragg et al., "Athlete Endorsements in Food Marketing," *Pediatrics* 132, no. 5 (July 2013), doi:10.1542/peds.2013-0093d (in 2010, 79 percent of athlete-endorsed foods were energy-dense and nutrient-poor, while almost 94 percent of athlete-endorsed drinks derived all of their calories from added sugar.)

75    *a 2018 study found that 76 percent of the products endorsed by leagues* Marie A. Bragg et al., "Sports Sponsorships of Food and Nonalcoholic Beverages," *Pediatrics* 141, no. 4 (2018), doi:10.1542/peds.2017-2822.

76    *even parents mistakenly believe a product is healthier when it's endorsed by an athlete* Helen Dixon et al., "Parents' Responses to Nutrient Claims and Sports Celebrity Endorsements on Energy-Dense and Nutrient-Poor Foods: an Experimental Study," *Public Health Nutrition* 14, no. 6 (October 2011): 1071–79, doi:10.1017/s1368980010003691.

76    *"but a character, even a friend"* Dulcie Leimbach, "Where Ads Aimed at Kids Come to Life," *New York Times*, December 13, 2000, www.nytimes.com/2000/12/13/business/marketing-where-ads-aimed-at-kids-come-to-life.html.

76    *a 2018 survey found that 95 percent of teens own a smartphone* Pew Research Center, "Teens, Social Media & Technology 2018," May 2018, http://www.pewinternet.org/2018/05/31/teens-social-media-technology-2018/.

76    *nearly half of these children already own their own tablet device* Common Sense Media, "The Common Sense Census: Media Use by Kids Age Zero to Eight," 2017, https://www.commonsensemedia.org/sites/default/files/uploads/research/0-8_executivesummary_release_final_1.pdf.

76    *she receives a friendly tweet from Red Bull* https://twitter.com/redbull/status/999400680031911936.

77    *blind taste test of twenty-five kinds of Pringles* It's unclear whether this Pringles video was sponsored by the brand, but it's notable that Evan YouTube (as he's called) is affiliated with a company that connects YouTube influencers to brands. He also has a spotty record of disclosing his corporate ties ("'Evan YouTube' YouTube Channels to Disclose Sponsored Videos as Advertising Following CARU Inquiry," September 12, 2016, http://www.asrcreviews.org/evantube-youtube-channels-to-disclose-sponsored-videos-as-advertising-following-caru-inquiry/). For more on how brands capitalize on child YouTube stars, see Sapna Maheshwari, "Online and Making Thousands,

at Age 4: Meet the Kidfluencers," *New York Times*, March 1, 2019, https://www.nytimes.com/2019/03/01/business/media/social-media-influencers-kids.html.

77  *he's told that water, unlike sugar-sweetened Gatorade, is the "enemy" of athletic performance* Nancy Huehnergarth, "Water Is the Enemy, Gatorade Mobile Game Tells Youth," *Civil Eats*, January 13, 2014, civileats.com/2014/01/07/water-is-the-enemy-gatorade-mobile-game-tells-youth/. Writer and advocate Huehnergarth brought the game to the attention of the New York State Attorney General, which led to a settlement in which Gatorade agreed to removed the game from the Internet and pay $100,000 to the Partnership for a Healthier America's Drink Up! Initiative—a program which encourages kids to drink more water. See Nancy Huehnergarth, "Gatorade's 'War on Water' Dampened by NY Attorney General," Nancy F. Huehnergarth Consulting, October 26, 2014, nfhconsulting.com/2014/10/26/gatorades-war-on-water-dampened-by-ny-attorney-general/.

77  *Snapchat lens…will have garnered 224 million views* Sig Ueland, "10 Brands on Snapchat, for Innovative Marketing," *Practical Ecommerce*, February 15, 2017, www.practicalecommerce.com/10-Brands-on-Snapchat-for-Innovative-Marketing.

78  *today's kids still see about ten to eleven food-related commercials a day* Jennifer L. Harris et al., "FACTS 2017: Food Industry Self-Regulation After 10 Years: Progress and Opportunities to Improve Food Advertising to Children," UConn Rudd Center for Food Policy & Obesity (November 2017), http://www.uconnruddcenter.org/files/Pdfs/FACTS-2017_Final.pdf.

78  *Even kids' extracurricular activities aren't safe from marketers' reach* Bettina Elias Siegel, "Gatorade G Force Infiltrates High Schools Under the Guise of 'Hydration Education,'" *The Lunch Tray*, August 20, 2015, https://www.thelunchtray.com/gatorade-g-force-infiltrates-high-schools-under-guise-of-hydration-education/; Bragg et al., "Sports Sponsorships of Food and Nonalcoholic Beverages."

78  *Unhealthy food and beverage marketing creeps into children's lives in more subtle ways* Jennifer L. Harris, Kelly D. Brownell,

and John A. Bargh, "The Food Marketing Defense Model: Integrating Psychological Research to Protect Youth and Inform Public Policy," *Social Issues and Policy Review* 3, no. 1 (2009): 211–71, at 213, doi:10.1111/j.1751-2409.2009.01015.x.

78  *"surround marketing"* Janice Rosenberg, "Brand Loyalty Begins Early," *Ad Age*, February 12, 2001, https://adage.com/article/interactive/brand-loyalty-begins-early/55486/.

78  *"You've got to become part of the fabric of their lives"* Ad executive quote found at Consumers Union, "Selling America's Kids: Commercial Pressures on Kids of the 90's," https://consumersunion.org/news/selling-americas-kids-commercial-pressures-on-kids-of-the-90s-part-one/.

78  *has also found that this desire can be instilled with as little as one commercial exposure* Behnam Sadeghirad et al., "Influence of Unhealthy Food and Beverage Marketing on Children's Dietary Intake and Preference: A Systematic Review and Meta-Analysis of Randomized Trials," *Obesity Reviews* 17, no. 10 (2016): 945–59, doi:10.1111/obr.12445; Brian L. Wilcox et al., "Report of the APA Task Force on Advertising and Children," American Psychological Association, February 20, 2004, https://www.apa.org/pi/families/resources/advertising-children.pdf.

79  *fewer than 10 percent advertised healthier foods like yogurt, water, etc.* Jennifer L. Harris et al., "FACTS 2017: Food Industry Self-Regulation After 10 Years."

79  *kids of color get a double dose of this unhealthy food marketing* "Increasing Disparities in Unhealthy Food Advertising Targeted to Hispanic and Black Youth," a report by the UConn Rudd Center for Food Policy & Obesity, Council on Black Health, and Salud America!, January, 2019, http://uconnruddcenter.org/files/Pdfs/TargetedMarketingReport2019.pdf; Punam Ohri-Vachaspati et al., "Child-Directed Marketing Inside and on the Exterior of Fast Food Restaurants," *American Journal of Preventive Medicine* 48, no. 1 (2015): 22–30, doi:10.1016/j.amepre.2014.08.011.

79  *Those who saw food ads ate 45 percent more Goldfish than kids who'd seen non-food ads* Jennifer L. Harris, John A. Bargh, and

Kelly D. Brownell, "Priming Effects of Television Food Advertising on Eating Behavior," *Health Psychology* 28, no. 4 (2009): 404–13, doi:10.1037/a0014399.

79   *a 2018 study in the UK found that when kids saw Instagram posts of popular celebrities* "YouTube Stars 'Might Encourage Kids to Eat More Calories,'" *BBC News*, May 26, 2018, https://www.bbc.com/news/health-44258509.

79   *a 2015 analysis of forty-five different priming studies* Rebecca G. Boswell and Hedy Kober, "Food Cue Reactivity and Craving Predict Eating and Weight Gain: A Meta-Analytic Review," *Obesity Reviews* 17, no. 2 (August 2015): 159–77, doi:10.1111/obr.12354.

79   *moms collectively resorted to ten different strategies to deal with nagging* Henry and Borzekowski, "The Nag Factor."

79   *nagging usually takes place in public* Cara Wilking, "Issue Brief: Reining in Pester Power Food and Beverage Marketing," The Public Health Advocacy Institute, September 2011, http://www.phaionline.org/wp-content/uploads/2011/09/Pester_power.pdf.

80   *Pester Power causes a "high level of frustration and stress" for parents* Henry and Borzekowski, "The Nag Factor."

80   *marketing anything to children in this age group is inherently unfair and deceptive* Brian L. Wilcox et al., "Report of the APA Task Force on Advertising and Children," American Psychological Association, February 20, 2004, https://www.apa.org/pi/families/resources/advertising-children.pdf; "Perspectives on Marketing, Self-Regulation and Childhood Obesity," Federal Trade Commission Workshop remarks by Donald Shifrin, member, AAP Task Force on Obesity and chair, AAP Committee on Communications, July 14–15, 2005, Washington, DC, https://www.aap.org/en-us/advocacy-and-policy/federal-advocacy/Pages/Perspectives-on-Marketing,-Self-Regulation-and-Childhood-Obesity.aspx; McGinnis, *Food Marketing to Children and Youth: Threat or Opportunity?*

80   *one study found only 40 percent of kids aged eleven to twelve truly understood* Jennifer L. Harris, Amy Heard, and

Marlene B. Schwartz, "Older But Still Vulnerable: All Children Need Protection From Unhealthy Food Marketing," Yale (now UConn) Rudd Center for Food Policy & Obesity policy brief, January 2014, accessed at http://www.uconnruddcenter.org/files/Pdfs/Protecting_Older_Children_3_14.pdf.

80  *like the product placements woven into video games, movies, etc.* See the studies cited in ibid.

80  *a 2015 Rudd Center survey found that 85 percent of parents* Jennifer L. Harris, Karen S. Haraghey, Yoon-Young Choi, and Frances Fleming-Milici, "Parents' Attitudes About Food Marketing to Children—2012 to 2015: Opportunities and Challenges to Creating Demand For a Healthier Food Environment," UConn Rudd Center for Food Policy & Obesity (April 2017), http://www.uconnruddcenter.org/ParentAttitudes.

81  *A 1979 ABC News poll found that 79 percent of the public supported a ban on advertising* Michael Pertschuk, *Revolt Against Regulation: the Rise and Pause of the Consumer Movement* (Oakland: University of California Press, 1982), 49.

81  *"junk food" advertisers against the health and well-being of the American child and family"* Pertschuk, *Revolt Against Regulation,* 70–71.

82  *"there was no way we could win"* Ibid., 71.

82  *"It is not a journey that anyone at the commission cares to repeat"* J. Howard Beales III, "Advertising to Kids and the FTC: A Regulatory Retrospective That Advises the Present," based on a speech delivered by Beales, then the director of the FTC's Bureau of Consumer Protection, to the George Mason Law Review 2004 Symposium on Antitrust and Consumer Protection, accessed at https://www.ftc.gov/sites/default/files/documents/public_statements/advertising-kids-and-ftc-regulatory-retrospective-advises-present/040802adstokids.pdf.

82  *The report also specifically cited child-directed food and beverage advertising* Catharyn T. Liverman et al., *Preventing Childhood Obesity: Health in the Balance* (Washington, DC: National Academies Press, 2005).

83    contributing to "an environment that puts their health at risk"
      McGinnis, *Food Marketing to Children and Youth: Threat or
      Opportunity?*

83    *if they didn't, "Congress should enact legislation"* Ibid., 14–15.

83    *(CFBAI), which is dedicated to voluntarily improving child-
      directed food and drink advertising* CFBAI, "Changing the
      Landscape of Food & Beverage Advertising: The Children's
      Food & Beverage Advertising Initiative in Action—A Progress
      Report on the First Six Months of Implementation: July–
      December 2007," https://www.bbb.org/us/storage/0/Shared%
      20Documents/CFBAI%20Report.pdf.

83    *each has pledged to: only market "healthier dietary choices" to
      kids under twelve* In 2018, CFBAI's eighteen participants were:
      American Licorice Company; Burger King Corporation;
      Campbell Soup Company; The Coca-Cola Company; Conagra
      Brands, Inc.; Danone North America; PBC, Ferrero USA, Inc.;
      General Mills, Inc.; The Hershey Company; Kellogg Company;
      The Kraft Heinz Company; Mars, Incorporated; McDonald's
      USA; Mondelez Global, LLC; Nestlé USA; PepsiCo, Inc.;
      Post Foods, LLC; and Unilever USA. The CFBAI's core
      principles may be found at "Children's Food and Beverage
      Advertising Initiative Program and Core Principles Statement,
      4th edition," https://bbbprograms.org/siteassets/documents/
      cfbai/enhanced-core-principles-fourth-edition-with-
      appendix-a.pdf.

83    *resulting in approved product lists that included...* See, e.g.,
      CFBAI, "Changing the Landscape of Food & Beverage
      Advertising," Appendix C. The CFBAI posts yearly compliance
      reports, including current approved product lists, at https://
      bbbprograms.org/programs/CFBAI/cfbai-compliance--
      progress-reports/.

83    *one dismayed parent asked, "If these are the better-for-you foods,
      what's the worst list?"* Amy E. Ustjanauskas et al., "Focus Groups
      with Parents: What Do They Think about Food Marketing to
      Their Kids?" Yale (now UConn) Rudd Center for Food Policy &

Obesity (May 2010) http://www.uconnruddcenter.org/files/ Pdfs/RuddReport_FocusGroupsParents_5_10.pdf.

83  *pledge only applies to advertising on "child-directed" media.... the definition should be expanded to include children under fifteen* Jennifer L. Harris, Vishnudas Sarda, Marlene B. Schwartz, and Kelly D. Brownell, "Redefining 'Child-Directed Advertising' to Reduce Unhealthy Television Food Advertising," *American Journal of Preventive Medicine* 44, no. 4 (2013), doi:10.1016/s0749-3797(13)00125-6; Healthy Eating Research, *Recommendations for Responsible Food Marketing to Children*, January 2015, http://healthyeatingresearch.org/wp-content/uploads/2015/01/ HER_Food-Marketing-Recomm_1-2015.pdf.

84  *if you happen to read the footnotes on its pledge* "Children's Food and Beverage Advertising Initiative Program and Core Principles Statement, 4th edition," footnote 8, https://bbbprograms.org/ siteassets/documents/cfbai/enhanced-core-principles-fourth-edition-with-appendix-a.pdf.

84  *Ads for fruits and vegetables accounted for less than one percent of all CFBAI advertising* Dale Kunkel, Christopher McKinley, and Paul Wright, "The Impact of Industry Self-Regulation on the Nutritional Quality of Foods Advertised on Television to Children," report commissioned by Children Now (December 2009) http://lahealthaction.org/library/adstudy09_report. pdf.

85  *Congress directed four federal agencies...to come up with a stronger set of nutrition standards* Omnibus Appropriations Act, 2009, HR 1105, 111th Cong., Congressional Record 155, pt. 4: 4831.

85  *"Are we doing everything that we can to secure the health and future of our kids?"* The White House Archives of President Barack Obama, Office of the First Lady, "Remarks by the First Lady at a Grocery Manufacturers Association Conference," March 16, 2010, https://obamawhitehouse.archives.gov/the-press-office/remarks-first-lady-a-grocery-manufacturers-association-conference.

85    *food and beverage companies knew they had to do better* The proposed IWG guidelines may be found at https://www.ftc .gov/news-events/press-releases/2011/04/interagency-working-group-seeks-input-proposed-voluntary.

85    *The coalition claimed the guidelines would somehow kill 400,000 jobs, result in $152 billion in lost revenue* "Important New Data Clearly Show Impact of Proposed IWG Guidelines on Fragile Economic Recovery," *ANA*, www.ana.net/content/show/ id/21700; Marion Nestle, "Help! Rescue the Government's Marketing-to-Kids Nutrition Standards!" *Food Politics*, October 9, 2011, www.foodpolitics.com/2011/09/help-rescue-the -governments-marketing-to-kids-nutrition-standards/.

85    *lobbying dollars flowed in by the millions to sway key legislators* Duff Wilson and Janet Roberts, "Special Report: How Washington Went Soft on Childhood Obesity," *Reuters*, April 27, 2012, www.reuters.com/article/us-usa-foodlobby/special-report -how-washington-went-soft-on-childhood-obesity -idUSBRE83Q0ED20120427. According to Reuters, between 2009 and 2012, the food and beverage industries more than doubled their prior lobbying expenditures to combat various Obama administration efforts to improve public health, including the IWG.

86    *neither the First Lady nor anyone else from the White House spoke up* Wilson and Roberts, "Special Report." A White House spokesman told Reuters the Obama administration "consistently supported" the IWG, but "could not point to any specific example of the president or First Lady voicing support" for it.

86    *a special Reuters report shed light on what had really gone down* Wilson and Roberts, "Special Report."

86    *"I'd focus more on exercise, too, if my husband was up for re-election"* Wilson and Roberts, "Special Report."

86    *"It's hard to believe how thoroughly Congress is in bed with the food industry"* Marion Nestle, "Congress Caves in Again, Delays IWG Recommendations," *Food Politics*, December 10, 2011, www.foodpolitics.com/2011/12/congress-caves-in-again-delays-iwg-recommendations/; Marion Nestle, "Let's Move Campaign Gives up on Healthy Diets for Kids?" *Food Politics*,

February 4, 2012, www.foodpolitics.com/2011/12/lets-move-campaign-gives-up-on-healthy-diets-for-kids/.

87 *"When it comes to kids' health, they shouldn't go wobbly in the knees"* Wilson and Roberts, "Special Report."

87 *CFBAI formally adopted uniform standards to apply across the board* CFBAI's uniform nutrition standards may be accessed at https://bbbprograms.org/siteassets/documents/cfbai/cfbai-category-specific-uniform-nutrition-criteria.pdf.

87 *Examples from CFBAI's 2018 approved product list include* CFBAI's 2018 approved product list may be accessed at https://bbbprograms.org/contentassets/bec09ff757ca4201b699ceac4f28a7a1/cfbai-product-list-july-2018.pdf.

87 *can't legally be sold in public schools due to their excessive calories, sugar, and/or fat* Jennifer L. Harris et al., "FACTS 2017: Food Industry Self-Regulation After 10 Years: Progress and Opportunities to Improve Food Advertising to Children," UConn Rudd Center for Food Policy & Obesity (November 2017), http://www.uconnruddcenter.org/files/Pdfs/FACTS-2017_Final.pdf.

87 *the IWG's own description of what its guidelines were meant to achieve* Federal Trade Commission, "Interagency Working Group Seeks Input on Proposed Voluntary Principles for Marketing Food to Children," press release, April 28, 2011, https://www.ftc.gov/news-events/press-releases/2011/04/interagency-working-group-seeks-input-proposed-voluntary. A complete description of the IWG's proposed principles may be found at Interagency Working Group on Food Marketed to Children, "Preliminary Proposed Nutrition Principles to Guide Industry Self-Regulatory Efforts, Request for Comments," April 28, 2011, https://www.ftc.gov/sites/default/files/documents/public_events/food-marketed-children-forum-interagency-working-group-proposal/110428foodmarketproposedguide.pdf.

88 *kids are still seeing, on average, three television commercials a day* Harris et al., "FACTS 2017: Food Industry Self-Regulation After 10 Years," 8.

88 *appeared to be directly targeting young teens* Harris et al., "FACTS 2017: Food Industry Self-Regulation After 10 Years," 9.

89    *"at least until their own kids start making requests"* Press
      release, *Packaged Facts: Three Mega Trends Impacting Kids Food
      Industry*, March 31, 2016, https://www.packagedfacts.com/
      about/release.asp?id=3879.

## 5. Cafeteria Copycats

91    *elementary schools of Appling County, Georgia* Appling County
      School District (Baxley, Georgia) September 2018 menu
      accessed at http://www.appling.k12.ga.us/view/13420.pdf.

91    *elementary school entrées in Grosse Pointe, Michigan* Grosse
      Pointe Public Schools September 2018 menu accessed at
      https://gpschools.nutrislice.com/menu/defer/lunch/2018-
      09-19.

92    *Many districts . . . had to make their school meals look more
      like junk food* Janet Poppendieck, *Free for All: Fixing School
      Food in America* (Berkeley: University of California Press,
      2010), 64–76.

92    *Veggie Wrap was forced to duke it out with the Crispy Corn Dog*
      St. Louis Public Schools menu accessed at https://saintlouisps.
      nutrislice.com.

92    *"Top 10 Worst Fast Food Meal"* Sean Gregory and Kristi
      Oloffson, "Top 10 Worst Fast-Food Meals," *Time*, June 18, 2009,
      http://content.time.com/time/specials/packages/article/
      0,28804,1905549_1905546_1905486,00.html.

93    *As of 2016, Domino's was reportedly providing Smart Slice to
      over six thousand districts* Judy Hall, "Why the Dairy Checkoff
      Partnered with Domino's," *Progressive Dairyman*, May 6, 2016,
      https://www.progressivedairy.com/news/organizations/why-
      the-dairy-checkoff-partnered-with-domino-s.

93    *Michelle Obama was frequently mocked as a member of the Food
      Police* Shauna Theel, "Right-Wing Media Attack Michelle
      Obama for Fighting Childhood Obesity," *Media Matters for
      America*, September 17, 2010, https://www.mediamatters.org/
      research/2010/09/17/right-wing-media-attack-michelle-
      obama-for-figh/170761.

94  *a comprehensive 2019 study commissioned by the U.S. Department of Agriculture* Mary Kay Fox et al., "School Nutrition and Meal Cost Study," U.S. Department of Agriculture, Food and Nutrition Service, Office of Policy Support, Final Report Volume 4: Student Participation, Satisfaction, Plate Waste, and Dietary Intakes, 53, 78, https://fns-prod.azureedge.net/sites/default/files/resource-files/SNMCS-Volume4.pdf (finding that rates of student participation were "significantly higher" at schools where lunches scored higher on the Healthy Eating Index; finding that plate waste measurements from over 6,000 lunch trays at 165 schools in the 2014-2015 school year were found to be "generally comparable to findings from studies that examined plate waste prior to implementation of the updated nutrition standards"). The USDA's plate waste finding was consistent with two earlier, well-designed plate waste studies: Juliana F.W. Cohen et al., "Impact of the New U.S. Department of Agriculture School Meal Standards on Food Selection, Consumption, and Waste," *American Journal of Preventive Medicine* 46, no. 4 (April 2014): 388–94, doi:10.1016/j.amepre.2013.11.013; Marlene B. Schwartz et al., "New School Meal Regulations Increase Fruit Consumption and Do Not Increase Total Plate Waste," *Childhood Obesity* 11, no. 3 (June 1, 2015): 242–47, doi:10.1089/chi.2015.0019.

94  *decades-long efforts of public health advocates* Colin Schwartz and Margo G. Wootan, "How a Public Health Goal Became a National Law," *Nutrition Today*, 2019, 1, doi:10.1097/nt.0000000000000318.

94  *there's still no limit on the amount of added sugar that can be served to kids* This omission relates specifically to the federally subsidized school meal. Under the HHFKA, so-called "competitive" foods and beverages—those sold in the cafeteria's à la carte snack line as well as in school stores, vending machines, and via fundraisers—can have no more than 35 percent sugar by weight. But that's still a significant amount.

94  *most districts rely heavily on cheaper grain entrées like cereals, muffins, etc.* Bettina Elias Siegel, "Why There Is So Much Sugar in Your Kid's School Breakfast," *Civil Eats*, December 3, 2016,

https://civileats.com/2015/09/24/why-there-is-so-much-sugar-in-your-kids-school-breakfast/.

95 *juice and fruit aren't interchangeable, due to juice's relative lack of fiber and high concentration of free sugar* Ibid.; Erika R. Cheng, Lauren G. Fiechtner, and Aaron E. Carroll, "Seriously, Juice Is Not Healthy," *New York Times*, July 7, 2018, https://www.nytimes.com/2018/07/07/opinion/sunday/juice-is-not-healthy-sugar.html; "The Science Behind the Sweetness in Our Diets," *Bulletin of the World Health Organization* 92, no. 11 (2014): 780–81, doi:10.2471/blt.14.031114.

95 *elementary school student in Broward County, Florida* Heron Heights Elementary (Broward County Public Schools) September 2018 breakfast menu accessed at https://schools.mealviewer.com/school/HeronHeightsElementarySchool.

95 *A child in Stamford, Connecticut* Stamford Public Schools September 2018 elementary school breakfast menu accessed at https://stamfordpublicschools.nutrislice.com.

96 *you have a purchaser for life* See, e.g., Sam Oches, "School's in Session for Quick Serves," *QSR Magazine*, March 26, 2012, https://www.qsrmagazine.com/consumer-trends/school-s-session-quick-serves, quoting an industry member saying, "If I'm trying to influence a child and really grow my brand, the fact that I would be able to serve in a school helps my brand equity."

97 *Their aggressive lobbying campaign... crushed the proposal* Jen Lynds, "Obama Strikes down Proposed Limitation on Potatoes in School Meals," *Bangor Daily News*, November 18, 2011, https://bangordailynews.com/2011/11/18/news/aroostook/obama-strikes-down-proposed-limitation-on-potatoes-in-school-meals/.

97 *their dried fruit wouldn't make the cut due to its high sugar content* Larry Bivins, "Cranberry Industry Wary of Upcoming Nutrition Standards," *USA Today*, June 24, 2012, https://usatoday30.usatoday.com/news/nation/story/2012-06-24/cranberry-nutrition-standards/55795734/1#mainstory.

97 *Minnesota Senator Amy Klobuchar led the fight to preserve the loophole* David Rogers, "Potato Politics, with a Pizza Side,"

*POLITICO*, November 12, 2011, https://www.politico.com/ story/2011/11/potato-politics-with-a-pizza-side-068206.

97    **"It's not democracy, it's DiGiorno"** *The Daily Show with Jon Stewart*, November 16, 2011, http://www.cc.com/video-clips/ b0d7f6/the-daily-show-with-jon-stewart-superbad.

97    *Fully half of the organization's $10 million annual operating budget* Helena Bottemiller Evich, "Behind the School Lunch Fight," *POLITICO*, June 4, 2014, https://www.politico.com/ story/2014/06/michelle-obama-public-school-lunch-school-nutrition-association-lets-move-107390; School Nutrition Association 2018 Patron list accessed at https://schoolnutrition. org/uploadedFiles/Membership/Industry_Membership/ 2018-Patron-List.pdf.

98    *The Pillsbury Doughboy was on hand for photo ops* Kiera Butler, "Yes, Cheetos, Funnel Cake, and Domino's Are Approved School Lunch Items," *Mother Jones*, July 16, 2014, https://www. motherjones.com/environment/2014/07/school-lunch-conference-cheetos/.

98    *"letter of the law" food* I give credit for the excellent "letter of the law" descriptor to Scott Richardson, former director of research and strategic initiatives for Project Bread, now a doctoral student at Harvard studying public health nutrition.

98    *Richard B. Russell National School Lunch Act of 1946* Richard B. Russell National School Lunch Act, 42 U.S.C. §1751 (1946). The law's "Declaration of Policy" is found in Section 2.

99    *House Agriculture Committee report that same year* U.S. Congress, House, Committee on Agriculture Report, 79th Congress, June 4, 1946, quoted in Gordon W. Gunderson, "The National School Lunch Program: Background and Development— National School Lunch Act Approved," https://www.fns.usda. gov/nslp/history.

99    *often turned to pushcarts, local stores, and even enterprising school janitors for less-than-healthy meals* Poppendieck, *Free for All*, 68–69, 261; Susan Levine, *School Lunch Politics: The Surprising History of America's Favorite Welfare Program* (Princeton, NJ: Princeton University Press, 2011), 22.

99   *women's groups and other charities stepped in* It should be noted, however, that another, less worthy goal of this education effort was to "Americanize" the diets of recent immigrants by exposing their children to American-style school meals. See Levine, *School Lunch Politics* at 25–29; Harvey Levenstein, *Revolution at the Table* (Berkeley: University of California Press, 2003), 118–19.

99   *lessons in nutrition were being communicated "silently, to be sure, but effectively"* U.S. Department of Agriculture, *Farmer's Bulletin* 712 (March 1916), accessed via the Child Nutrition Archives, Institute of Child Nutrition, School of Applied Sciences at the University of Mississippi.

99   *their role in "teaching children what to eat"* Department of Education—City of New York, Division of Reference and Research, *School Lunches—New York City Elementary Schools* (1923), accessed via the Child Nutrition Archives, Institute of Child Nutrition, School of Applied Sciences at the University of Mississippi.

99   *keeping kids from the "dangers of food sold by corner groceries, etc."* Levine, *School Lunch Politics*, 33.

99   *here's the USDA again, in 1916: "Every time a child buys food…"* Federal Bureau of Education, *Farmer's Bulletin* 712 (1919) ("By means of [school meals], children may be taught food values and they become accustomed to eating the kinds of food they should have."), accessed via the Child Nutrition Archives, Institute of Child Nutrition, School of Applied Sciences at the University of Mississippi.

100   *"They don't even realize it's good for them"* Domino's video accessed at https://www.youtube.com/watch?v=IXFHbabmlFI.

101   *In 2018, that federal reimbursement ranged from 45 cents per lunch…* I've admittedly oversimplified things a bit for ease of discussion. For example, districts in Alaska, Hawaii, and Puerto Rico get additional federal funding because it's harder to source food there, and there are some other caveats as well. See "National School Lunch, Special Milk, and School Breakfast Programs, National Average Payments/Maximum Reimbursement Rates" 82 *Code of Federal Regulations* 35175-

35178 (July 28, 2017), https://www.federalregister.gov/ documents/2017/07/28/2017-15956/national-school-lunch- special-milk-and-school-breakfast-programs-national-average- paymentsmaximum.

101  *commodity food makes up about 15 to 20 percent of all the food served* U.S. Department of Agriculture, Food and Nutrition Service, "White Paper: USDA Foods in the National School Lunch Program," February 2016, https://fns-prod.azureedge .net/sites/default/files/fdd/NSLP-White-Paper.pdf.

101  *most districts have about a dollar and change left over for the food itself* The rate of federal reimbursement was already too low before the passage of the Healthy, Hunger-Free Kids Act, and it couldn't cover that law's mandate to serve healthier, and therefore often more expensive, food. So Congress agreed to provide an additional six cents per child per lunch to cover those new costs, an amount reflected in the figures I've provided here. But when the law was under debate, most experts determined that districts actually needed an additional ten cents to buy the healthier food.

102  *"They [students] see a box with a name on it, that's where they're going"* Bettina Elias Siegel, "Under Betti Wiggins, Houston ISD Signs $8 Million Contract for Domino's Smart Slice Pizza," *The Lunch Tray*, August 2, 2018, https://www.thelunchtray.com/ houston-isd-8-million-contract-for-dominos-smart-slice- pizza-betti-wiggins/.

103  *workarounds that were "expensive, inefficient, and unsustainable"* Pew Charitable Trusts, "States Need Updated School Kitchen Equipment," March 26, 2014, http://www.pewtrusts.org/en/ research-and-analysis/reports/2014/03/26/states-need- updated-school-kitchen-equipment-b; Bettina Elias Siegel, "For School Lunch, Are Kitchens as Important as Ingredients?" *Civil Eats*, April 14, 2016, https://civileats.com/2016/02/16/in-the- case-of-school-lunch-kitchens-might-be-as-important-as- ingredients/.

103  *the 2014 Pew report pegged districts' total school kitchen infrastructure needs at $5 billion nationwide* Siegel, "Are Kitchens as Important as Ingredients?"; Pew Charitable Trusts

and Robert Wood Johnson Foundation, "USDA's School Kitchen Grants Benefit Meal Programs and Students," June 2016, https://www.pewtrusts.org/-/media/assets/2016/06/usdas_school_kitchen_grants_benefit_meal_programs_and_students.pdf.

104 *commodity cheese, flour, and tomato paste wind up ... a ConAgra frozen pizza* Robert Wood Johnson Foundation, "Impact of Federal Commodity Programs on School Meal Nutrition," September 1, 2008, https://www.rwjf.org/en/library/research/2008/09/impact-of-federal-commodity-programs-on-school-meal-nutrition.html; J. Amy Dillard, "Sloppy Joe, Slop, Sloppy Joe: How USDA Commodities Dumping Ruined the National School Lunch Program," *Oregon Law Review* 87, no. 1 (2008): 221–58; Lucy Komisar, "School Lunches and the Food Industry," *New York Times*, December 3, 2011, https://www.nytimes.com/2011/12/04/opinion/sunday/school-lunches-and-the-food-industry.html.

104 *if they don't, the manufacturer, not the district, will pay any fines* Poppendieck, *Free for All*, 102–3.

106 *that many schools, especially those in lower-income neighborhoods, are ringed by fast food outlets* Erin Blakemore, "For Students In Low-Income Schools, Fast Food Always in Easy Reach," *Huffington Post*, January 17, 2017, https://www.huffingtonpost.com/entry/for-students-in-low-income-schools-fast-food-always-in-easy-reach_us_57a21698e4b0104052a09ea6.

107 *low-income schools are less likely to regularly offer salads* Lindsey Turnery, Punam Ohri-Vachaspati, Lisa Powell, and Frank J. Chaloupka, "Improvements and Disparities in Types of Foods and Milk Beverages Offered in Elementary School Lunches, 2006–2007 to 2013–2014," *Preventing Chronic Disease* 13 (2016), doi:10.5888/pcd13.150395.

108 *Salad Bars to Schools, a nonprofit* Salad Bars to Schools, http://www.saladbars2schools.org/; the school garden figure comes from the USDA's 2015 school garden census (the most recent to date), accessed at https://farmtoschoolcensus.fns.usda.gov/farm-school-works-make-gardens-grow.

## 6. Just One Treat

110 *the Oxford Dictionary defines a "treat"* OxfordDictionaries.com, https://en.oxforddictionaries.com/definition/treat.

110 *8 grams of sugar* All nutrition information in this chapter was drawn from companies' respective websites or, in the case of non-branded food, from the Nutrionix website, https://www .nutritionix.com/.

111 *"school-sponsored fundraisers such as bake sales"* Chelsea Rudman, "Fox's War on Nutrition Continues with Fake Bake Sale Outrage," *Media Matters for America*, December 6, 2010, https://www.mediamatters.org/blog/2010/12/06/foxs-war-on-nutrition-continues-with-fake-bake/174067.

111 *others have exploited [this loophole] to the fullest* Elizabeth Piekarz-Porter, Wanting Lin, Yadira Herrera, and Jamie F. Chriqui, "Smart Snacks Fundraiser Exemption State Policies," Institute for Health Research and Policy, June 1, 2017, https://www.ihrp.uic.edu/files/Fundraiser%20 Exemptions_1June17.pdf; Howard Fischer, "Junk Food Allowed at Schools for Fundraising," *Arizona Daily Sun*, April 2, 2015, http://azdailysun.com/news/local/education/junk-food-allowed-at-schools-for-fundraising/article_7e597b18-25cc-5b4f-9779-1aa4bc9e8f4d.html.

111 *the fines were seen as just the cost of doing business* Bettina Elias Siegel, "Dispatch From Houston: School Junk Food Sales Are Alive and Well," *The Lunch Tray*, April 7, 2016, http://www .thelunchtray.com/school-fundraisers-junk-food-illegal-sales/.

112 *Texas's "exempt days" rule allows this kind of junk food fundraising* Ibid.

112 *Recent articles in education journals...also indicate that the practice persists* See, e.g., Carla Bafile, "Reward Systems That Work: What to Give and When to Give It!" *Education World*, July 20, 2017, https://www.educationworld.com/a_curr/ curr301.shtml; Derek Newton, "Public Schools Actually Embrace Innovation—Five Examples of States, Districts Making Tech Work," *Huffington Post*, July 28, 2017, https://www

.huffingtonpost.com/entry/public-schools-actually-embrace-innovation-five-examples_us_59778371e4b0940189700d12. Many online teacher resources continue to include reward charts and worksheets promising food rewards such as ice cream parties. See, e.g., https://www.teacherspayteachers.com/Browse/Search:ice%20cream%20reward.

114 *"Just the novelty of candy being part of a lesson... is enough to hold the attention of most children"* Candy Math: How to Make Your Own Inexpensive Math Manipulatives Using Candy or Cereal, accessed at homeschoolfreebies.s3.amazonaws.com/candymath.pdf.

115 *a study came out claiming mint boosts attention* Tim Post, "Teachers Hope to Boost Test Scores with Fresh Air, Food, Mints," *Minnesota Public Radio News*, April 18, 2012, https://www.mprnews.org/story/2012/04/18/mca-boost.

115 *One elementary school was actually caffeinating its kids with Mountain Dew soda on testing days* Mackenzie Ryan, "School Stops Giving Mountain Dew to Students Before Tests," *USA Today*, April 24, 2014, https://www.usatoday.com/story/news/nation-now/2014/04/24/school-stops-serving-mountain-dew/8109807/.

115 *kids who participate in youth sports leagues typically eat more junk food than kids who don't* Toben F. Nelson et al., "Do Youth Sports Prevent Pediatric Obesity? A Systematic Review and Commentary," *Current Sports Medicine Reports* 10, no. 6 (2011): 360–70, doi:10.1249/jsr.0b013e318237bf74; Julie Deardorff, "Kids Who Play Sports Eat More Junk Food: Study," *Chicago Tribune*, February 28, 2012, http://www.chicagotribune.com/lifestyles/chi-youth-sports-do-they-prevent-obesity-20120224-story.html.

116 *The American Academy of Pediatrics says most kids don't... need any hydration other than water* American Academy of Pediatrics, "Kids Should Not Consume Energy Drinks, and Rarely Need Sports Drinks, Says AAP," https://www.aap.org/en-us/about-the-aap/aap-press-room/pages/kids-should-not-consume-energy-drinks,-and-rarely-need-sports-drinks,-says-aap.aspx.

116  *40 percent of parents still believe Gatorade is a healthy beverage for children* Christina R. Munsell et al., "Parents' Beliefs about the Healthfulness of Sugary Drink Options: Opportunities to Address Misperceptions," *Public Health Nutrition* 19, no. 1 (November 2015): 46–54, doi:10.1017/s1368980015000397.

116  *"you know, win or lose, they look forward [to it]"* Aaron Rafferty et al., "Parents Report Competing Priorities Influence Snack Choice in Youth Sports," *Journal of Nutrition Education and Behavior* 50, no. 10 (November–December 2018), doi:10.1016/j.jneb.2018.04.275.

116  *this same survey found that a least some parents* Ibid.

116  *even as she typically consumes between 300 and 500 calories* Nelson et al., "Do Youth Sports Prevent Pediatric Obesity?"

117  *[G]randparents spoke of holding certain 'privileges' and having the right to 'spoil' grandchildren"* Karin Eli et al., "A Question of Balance: Explaining Differences Between Parental and Grandparental Perspectives on Preschoolers Feeding and Physical Activity," *Social Science & Medicine* 154 (2016): 28–35, doi:10.1016/j.socscimed.2016.02.030; Kylie G. Young et al., "Influence of Grandparents on the Dietary Intake of Their 2–12-Year-Old Grandchildren: A Systematic Review," *Nutrition & Dietetics* 75, no. 3 (2018): 291–306, doi:10.1111/1747-0080.12411.

118  *almost half of all dry-cleaners now offer some kind of free food* Tim Burke, "In-Store 'Extras' Favored by More Than Half of Dry Cleaners, Survey Shows," *American Drycleaner*, May 12, 2016, https://americandrycleaner.com/articles/store-extras-favored-more-half-dry-cleaners-survey-shows.

119  *According to market research commissioned by Spangler* Spangler website, https://www.spanglercandy.com/files/assets/researchgiveaway-candy.pdf.

119  *diners leave higher tips when a restaurant bill is offered with a few candy mints* David B. Strohmetz et al., "Sweetening the Till: The Use of Candy to Increase Restaurant Tipping," *Journal of Applied Social Psychology* 32, no. 2 (2002): 300–309, doi:10.1111/j.1559-1816.2002.tb00216.x.

119  *42 percent of parents will return to those businesses as a result*
Spangler website, https://www.spanglercandy.com/files/assets/
researchgiveaway-candy.pdf.

120  *Here's the manifesto I quickly pounded out* The Lunch Tray's
"Food-in-the-Classroom Manifesto" is available for free
download at https://www.thelunchtray.com/the-lunch-trays-
food-in-the-classroom-manifesto/.

## 7. Bigger Than Obesity

123  *almost 60 percent of today's children will be … obese* Specifically,
Harvard researchers projected that children who were aged two
to nineteen in 2016 had a 57 percent chance of being obese by
age thirty-five. Zachary J. Ward et al., "Simulation of Growth
Trajectories of Childhood Obesity into Adulthood," *New
England Journal of Medicine* 377, no. 22 (2017): 2145–53,
doi:10.1056/nejmoa1703860.

123  *"even this bleak projection may underestimate the magnitude of
the problem"* David S. Ludwig, "Epidemic Childhood Obesity:
Not Yet the End of the Beginning," *Pediatrics* 141, no. 3 (2018),
doi:10.1542/peds.2017–4078.

124  *some evidence that weight may be affected by less obvious things
like antibiotic use, etc.* James Hamblin, "Are Antibiotics Making
People Larger?" *Atlantic*, December 22, 2015, https://www
.theatlantic.com/health/archive/2015/12/obesity-antibiotics-
microbiome/421344/; Jerrold J. Heindel, Retha Newbold, and
Thaddeus T. Schug, "Endocrine Disruptors and Obesity," *Nature
Reviews Endocrinology* 11, no. 11 (November 2015): 653–61,
doi:10.1038/nrendo.2015.163; Eleonora Ponterio and Lucio
Gnessi, "Adenovirus 36 and Obesity: An Overview," *Viruses* 7,
no. 7 (July 2015): 3719–40, doi:10.3390/v7072787.

124  *scientists can't always explain why some kids gain excess weight
while others don't* Perri Klass, "Do Parents Make Kids Fat?"
*New York Times*, January 8, 2018, https://www.nytimes
.com/2018/01/08/well/family/do-parents-make-kids-fat
.html.

125 *In 2010…91 percent of American kids were eating a diet classified as affirmatively poor* Donald M. Lloyd-Jones et al., "Defining and Setting National Goals for Cardiovascular Health Promotion and Disease Reduction," *Circulation* 121, no. 4 (2010): 586–613, doi:10.1161/circulationaha.109.192703; see also Julia Steinberger et al., "Cardiovascular Health Promotion in Children: Challenges and Opportunities for 2020 and Beyond," *Circulation* 34, no. 12 (August 11, 2016): e236–e255, doi:10. 1161/cir.0000000000000441.

125 *a more recent American Heart Association study of older kids* Unpublished dietary analysis provided to the author by the American Heart Association's Center for Healthy Metrics and Evaluation.

125 *around 60 percent of the country's diet currently comes from highly processed foods* Steele E. Martínez et al., "Ultra-Processed Foods and Added Sugars in the US Diet: Evidence From a Nationally Representative Cross-Sectional Study," *BMJ Open* 6, no. 3 (March 9, 2016): e009892, doi: 10.1136/ bmjopen-2015-009892; Centers for Disease Control and Prevention, "Vital Signs: Fruit and Vegetable Intake Among Children—United States, 2003–2010," August 8, 2014, https:// www.cdc.gov/mmwr/preview/mmwrhtml/mm6331a3.htm?s_ cid=mm6331a3_w; Scientific Report of the 2015 Dietary Guidelines Advisory Committee, Advisory Report to the Secretary of Health and Human Services and the Secretary of Agriculture, February 2015, health.gov/dietaryguidelines/2015-scientific-report/.

126 *According to the latest federal data, the top six sources of calories among kids aged two to eighteen* 2015 Dietary Guidelines Report.

126 *when babies begin eating more table food, nutrition starts to takes a nosedive* Victor Fulgoni, III and Sanjiv Agarwal, "NHANES Analysis of Total Fruit, Vegetable, Whole Grains, Added Sugars and Sodium in 0–24 Months, 2001–2012" (2016 poster presentation commissioned by Beech-Nut Nutrition); Ariana Eunjung Cha, "Americans' Junk Food Habits Start in

Toddler Years. At Age 1, We Eat Fries and Brownies—But Few Veggies," *Washington Post*, April 6, 2016, https://www .washingtonpost.com/news/to-your-health/wp/2016/04/06/ americans-junk-food-habits-start-in-the-toddler-years-potato-chips-fries-among-top-vegetables/; PR Newswire, "New Research Reveals Infants as Young as Nine Months Are Eating Diets Low in Vegetables and Whole Grains, Yet High in Sodium and Added Sugars," April 6, 2016, https://www.prnewswire.com/news-releases/new-research-reveals-infants-as-young-as-nine-months-are-eating-diets-low-in-vegetables-and-whole-grains-yet-high-in-sodium-and-added-sugars-300247118.html; Heather C. Hamner et al., "Food Consumption Patterns among U.S. Children from Birth to 23 Months of Age, 2009–2014," *Nutrients* 9, no. 9 (August 26, 2017): 942, doi:10.3390/nu9090942.

127 (*Experts say babies under age two shouldn't be consuming any added sugars.*) Miriam B. Vos, "Added Sugars and Cardiovascular Disease Risk in Children: A Scientific Statement From the American Heart Association," *Circulation* 135, no. 19 (May 9, 2017): e1017–e1034, doi:10.1161/CIR.0000000000000439.

127 [*Toddlers are*] *also now consuming over 9 teaspoons of added sugar a day* Fulgoni, "NHANES Analysis;" Hamner et al., "Food Consumption Patterns."

127 *babies who drink sugar-sweetened beverages on a daily basis... are more likely to be doing the same at age six* Catherine Saint Louis, "Childhood Diet Habits Set in Infancy, Studies Suggest," *New York Times*, September 2, 2014, https://www .nytimes.com/2014/09/02/health/childhood-diet-habits-set-in-infancy-studies-suggest.html; Liping Pan, Bettylou Sherry, and Ruowei Li, "The Association of Sugar-Sweetened Beverage Intake During Infancy With Sugar-Sweetened Beverage Intake at 6 Years of Age," *Pediatrics* 134, supplement no. 1 (September 2014): S56-S62, doi:10.1542/peds.2014-0646J; Kirsten A. Grimm, Sonia A. Kim, Amy L. Yaroch, and Kelley S. Scanlon, "Fruit and Vegetable Intake During Infancy and Early Childhood," *Pediatrics* 134, supplement no. 1 (September 2014): S63-S69, doi:10.1542/peds.2014-0646K.

127 *but according to federal data, it's kids who are consuming the most [sugar]* U.S. Department of Health and Human Services and U.S. Department of Agriculture, *2015–2020 Dietary Guidelines for Americans*, 8th Edition, December 2015, http://health.gov/dietaryguidelines/2015/guidelines/, Figure 2-9.

127 *since 2013, seven of the top eight product categories were sugary* Market research commissioned by the author in 2018 from GlobalData, PLC, owner of the Products Launch Analytics database.

128 *83 percent of snacks marketed for toddlers containing added sweeteners* UConn Rudd Center for Food Policy & Obesity, "Baby Food FACTS: Nutrition and Marketing of Baby and Toddler Food and Drinks," January 2017, http://www.uconnruddcenter.org/BabyFoodFACTS; Samuel Lalitha, Danna Ethan, Corey Hannah Basch, and Benny Samuel, "A Comparative Study of the Sodium Content and Calories from Sugar in Toddler Foods Sold in Low- and High-Income New York City Supermarkets," *Global Journal of Health Science* 6, no. 5 (May 7, 2014): 22–29, doi:10.5539/gjhs.v6n5p22; Lindsey Tanner, "CDC Study: Toddler Food Often Has Too Much Salt and Sugar," *Washington Post*, February 2, 2015, https://www.washingtonpost.com/national/health-science/cdc-study-toddler-food-often-has-too-much-salt-and-sugar/2015/02/01/a2bba35c-aa57-11e4-abe8-e1ef60ca26de_story.html?utm_term=.0be7b5be65d4 (citing Mary E. Cogswell et al., "Sodium and Sugar in Complementary Infant and Toddler Foods Sold in the United States," *Pediatrics*, [February 2, 2015], doi:10.1542/peds.2014–3251.)

128 *Yogurt…can contain more sugar per serving than a brownie* Julia Belluz and Javier Zarracina, "We Need to Call American Breakfast What It Often Is: Dessert," *Vox*, March 7, 2018, https://www.vox.com/2016/7/11/12128372/sugar-cereal-breakfast-nutrition-facts.

128 *research shows kids tend to eat twice as much cereal when it's sweetened* Jennifer L. Harris et al., "Effects of Serving High-Sugar Cereals on Children's Breakfast-Eating Behavior,"

*Pediatrics* 127, no. 1 (January 1, 2011): http://pediatrics. aappublications.org/content/127/1/71.

128 **Because they don't fill kids up, these beverages only add extra calories** Centers for Disease Control and Prevention, "Get the Facts: Sugar-Sweetened Beverages and Consumption," April 7, 2017, https://www.cdc.gov/nutrition/data-statistics/sugar-sweetened-beverages-intake.html.

128 **60 percent still drink at least one sweetened beverage** Sara N. Bleich, Kelsey A. Vercammen, Jonathan Wyatt Koma, and Zhonghe Li, "Trends in Beverage Consumption Among Children and Adults, 2003–2014," *Obesity* 26, no. 2 (2017): 432–41, doi:10.1002/oby.22056.

128 **parents with the least accurate grasp of foods' sugar content tended to have children with the highest BMI scores** Gretchen Reynolds, "Parents Aren't Good Judges of Their Kids' Sugar Intake," *New York Times*, July 19, 2018, https://www.nytimes.com/2018/07/19/well/parents-kids-sugar-food.html.

128 **around 10 teaspoons of naturally occurring sugar per serving** Erika R. Cheng, Lauren G. Fiechtner, and Aaron E. Carroll, "Seriously, Juice Is Not Healthy," *New York Times*, July 7, 2018, https://www.nytimes.com/2018/07/07/opinion/sunday/juice-is-not-healthy-sugar.html.

129 **American Academy of Pediatrics advises parents to not give any juice to babies under the age of one** AAP Press Release, "American Academy of Pediatrics Recommends No Fruit Juice For Children Under 1 Year," May 22, 2017, https://www.aap.org/en-us/about-the-aap/aap-press-room/Pages/American-Academy-of-Pediatrics-Recommends-No-Fruit-Juice-For-Children-Under-1-Year.aspx.

129 **four of their top ten fruits are consumed in the form of some type of juice** Fulgoni, "NHANES Analysis."

129 **By preschool, more than half of kids are drinking 10 ounces of juice a day** Cheng, Feichtner, and Carroll, "Seriously, Juice Is Not Healthy."

129 **It's also offered to families through WIC** Cheng, Feichtner, and Carroll, "Seriously, Juice Is Not Healthy."

130 *in the words of one candid restaurateur* Peter Applebome, "Setting the Table for Kids' Cuisine," *New York Times*, March 19, 1989, https://www.nytimes.com/1989/03/19/business/setting-the-table-for-kids-cuisine.html.

130 *Americans now spend more on food eaten outside the home* United States Department of Agriculture, Economic Research Service, "U.S. Food-Away-From-Home Spending Continued to Outpace At-Home Spending in 2017," https://www.ers.usda .gov/data-products/chart-gallery/gallery/chart-detail/?chartId=58364; Matt Phillips, "No One Cooks Anymore," *Quartz*, June 14, 2016, https://qz.com/706550/no-one-cooks-anymore/?utm_source=nextdraft&utm_medium=email.

130 *25 percent of kids' calories come from sources outside the home* Biing-Hwan Lin and Rosanna Mentzer Morrison, "Food and Nutrient Intake Data: Taking a Look at the Nutritional Quality of Foods Eaten at Home and Away From Home," U.S. Department of Agriculture, Economic Research Service, June 5, 2012, https://www.ers.usda.gov/amber-waves/2012/june/data-feature-food-and-nutrient-intake-data/.

130 *just over a third of children now eat fast food on any given day* Sundeep Vikraman, Cheryl D. Fryar, and Cynthia L. Ogden, "Caloric Intake from Fast Food Among Children and Adolescents in the United States, 2011–2012," Centers for Disease Control and Prevention, National Center for Health Statistics, September 2015, https://www.cdc.gov/nchs/products/databriefs/db213.htm.

130 *There have been improvements in recent years in the kids' side dishes offered by fast food chains* Megan P. Mueller et al., "Availability of Healthier Children's Menu Items in the Top Selling Quick Service Restaurant Chains (2004–2015)," *American Journal of Public Health* 109, no. 2 (2019): 267–69, doi:10.2105/ajph.2018.304800.

130 *eight major chains to date...have dropped sugary drinks...as the default beverage* Sara Ribakove, Jessica Almy, and Margo G. Wootan, "Soda on the Menu: Improvements Seen

But More Change Needed For Beverages On Restaurant Children's Menus," Center for Science in the Public Interest, July 2017, https://cspinet.org/kidsbeveragestudy.

130  *the majority of top chains (74 percent) still have sugary drinks on their children's menus* Ribakove, Almy, and Wootan, "Soda on the Menu."

130  *a 2016 study of the top two hundred restaurant chains* Deborah A. Cohen et al., "Kid's Menu Portion Sizes," *Nutrition Today* 51, no. 6 (2016): 273–80, doi:10.1097/nt.0000000000000179.

130  *A key driver of those excess calories is portion size* Cohen et al., "Kids' Menu Portion Sizes."

130  *when young children were offered an entrée twice the appropriate portion size* Jennifer Orlet Fisher, Barbara J. Rolls, and Leann L. Birch, "Children's Bite Size and Intake of an Entrée Are Greater with Large Portions than with Age-appropriate or Self-selected Portions," *American Journal of Clinical Nutrition* 77, no. 5 (2003): 1164-170, doi:10.1093/ajcn/77.5.1164.

131  *pizza is itself a significant contributor to the childhood obesity epidemic* Lisa M. Powell, Binh T. Nguyen, William H. Dietz, "Energy and Nutrient Intake From Pizza in the United States," *Pediatrics* 135, no. 2 (2015), doi:10.1542/peds.2014-1844d.

132  *25 million Americans will have [fatty liver] disease by 2025* Anahad O'Connor, "Threat Grows From Liver Illness Tied to Obesity," *New York Times*, June 13, 2014, https://well.blogs.nytimes.com/2014/06/13/threat-grows-from-liver-illness-tied-to-obesity/.

131  *a poor diet may undermine cognition* Michelle D. Florence, Mark Asbridge, and Paul J. Veugelers, "Diet Quality and Academic Performance," *Journal of School Health* 78, no. 4 (April 2008): 209–15, doi:10.1111/j.1746-1561.2008.00288.x; F. Gómez-Pinilla, "Brain Foods: The Effects of Nutrients on Brain Function," *Nature Reviews Neuroscience* 9, no. 7 (August 2008): 568–78, doi:10.1038/nrn2421; Barilla Center for Food and Nutrition, "Unhealthy Food Goes to Your Head," https://www.barillacfn.com/en/magazine/food-and-health/

unhealthy-food-goes-to-your-head/; Amy C. Reichelt, "Adolescent Maturational Transitions in the Prefrontal Cortex and Dopamine Signaling as a Risk Factor for the Development of Obesity and High Fat/High Sugar Diet Induced Cognitive Deficits," *Frontiers in Behavioral Neuroscience* 10 (October 13, 2016), doi:10.3389/fnbeh.2016.00189.

133 *In 1999, Ludwig and his colleagues divided twelve obese teen boys into three groups* David S. Ludwig et al., "High Glycemic Index Foods, Overeating, and Obesity," *Pediatrics* 103, no. 3 (March 1999): E26, doi: 10.1542/peds.103.3.e26.

134 *In a fascinating 2013 study, Ludwig's team gave twelve obese men milkshakes* B. S. Lennerz et al., "Effects of Dietary Glycemic Index on Brain Regions Related to Reward and Craving in Men," *American Journal of Clinical Nutrition* 98, no. 3 (September 2013): 641–47, doi:10.3945/ajcn.113.064113.

134 *including an increased risk of anxiety or depression* Adrienne O'Neil et al., "Relationship Between Diet and Mental Health in Children and Adolescents: A Systematic Review," *American Journal of Public Health* 104, no. 10 (2014), doi:10.2105/ajph.2014.302110.

134 *stress . . . can increase people's cravings for junk food* Walter C. Willett, "How Stress Can Make Us Overeat," *Harvard Health* blog, www.health.harvard.edu/healthbeat/how-stress-can-make-us-overeat.

134 *When researchers had a group of teenagers sleep just six hours a night* Dean W. Beebe et al., "Dietary Intake Following Experimentally Restricted Sleep in Adolescents," *Sleep* 36, no. 6 (June 1, 2013): 827–34, doi:10.5665/sleep.2704.

135 *kids more likely than adults to develop diabetes-related complications* Denise Grady, "Obesity-Linked Diabetes in Children Resists Treatment," *New York Times*, April 29, 2012, https://www.nytimes.com/2012/04/30/health/research/obesity-and-type-2-diabetes-cases-take-toll-on-children.html.

135 *[obesity is] believed to be the second most important risk factor for cancer* Mika Kivimäki et al., "Body Mass Index and Risk of Dementia: Analysis of Individual-Level Data from 1.3 Million

Individuals," *Alzheimer's & Dementia* 14, no. 5 (May 2018): 601–19, doi:10.1016/j.jalz.2017.09.016; Caitlin Dow, "Extra Pounds Means Extra Cancer Risk," *Nutrition Action*, March 30, 2018, https://www.nutritionaction.com/daily/diet-and-weight-loss/extra-pounds-means-extra-cancer-risk/.

136 *One recent study even found that being bullied as a teen correlates with obesity* Rebecca M. Puhl et al., "Experiences of Weight Teasing in Adolescence and Weight-Related Outcomes in Adulthood: A 15-year Longitudinal Study," *Preventive Medicine* 100 (2017): 173–79, doi:10.1016/j.ypmed.2017.04.023.

136 *overweight and obese kids face an increased risk of depression, anxiety, etc.* Amy Roeder, "The Scarlet F," *Harvard Public Health*, July 31, 2017, www.hsph.harvard.edu/magazine/magazine_article/the-scarlet-f/; Rebecca M. Puhl, "Childhood Obesity and Stigma," *Obesity Action Coalition*, http://www.obesityaction.org/educational-resources/resource-articles-2/childhood-obesity-resource-articles/childhood-obesity-and-stigma.

137 *Eleanor's experience wasn't unusual, according to researchers* Asheley Cockrell Skinner, "Parental Recall of Doctor Communication of Weight Status," *Archives of Pediatrics & Adolescent Medicine* 166, no. 4 (2012): 317, doi:10.1001/archpediatrics.2011.1135.

137 *guidance to help doctors navigate these potentially sensitive discussions* Neville H. Golden, Marcie Schneider, and Christine Wood, "Preventing Obesity and Eating Disorders in Adolescents," *Pediatrics* 138, no. 3 (2016), doi:10.1542/peds.2016-1649.

137 *he's statistically more likely to become an overweight or obese adult* Solveig A. Cunningham, Michael R. Kramer, and K. M. Venkat Narayan, "Incidence of Childhood Obesity in the United States," *New England Journal of Medicine* 370, no. 5 (January 30, 2014): 403–11, doi:10.1056/NEJMoa1309753.

138 *"Yet that parent of today is far more likely to be obese and/or diabetic"* David L. Katz, "My Conversation with Michael Moss: Bullies, Bodies, and the Body Politic," *Huffington Post*, March 1, 2013, https://www.huffpost.com/entry/food-industry-health_b_2775984.

139 *"The modern food era has spread out a smorgasbord of hyper-palatable...foods"* Madeline Drexler, ed., "Obesity: Can We Stop the Epidemic?" *Harvard Public Health Magazine*, June 13, 2017, https://www.hsph.harvard.edu/magazine/magazine_article/obesity/.

139 *"The food industry brings in serious muscle to bully us..."* Katz, "My Conversation with Michael Moss."

139 *"By the time weight piles up in adulthood, it's usually too late."* Drexler, "Obesity: Can We Stop the Epidemic?"

## 8. Pushing Back

141 *LFTB is made from slaughterhouse scraps* Michael Moss, "Safety of Beef Processing Method Is Questioned," *New York Times*, December 31, 2009, https://www.nytimes.com/2009/12/31/us/31meat.html.

142 **540 Meals appeared to be McDonald's decade-too-late rebuttal** *540 Meals: Choices Make the Difference*, accessed at https://www.youtube.com/watch?v=jxY9CAftk14.

143 *Cisna says in an earlier self-published book,* **My McDonald's Diet,** *that he hatched the plan over dinner with a friend* John Cisna and Ed Sweet, *My McDonald's Diet: How I Lost 37 Pounds in 90 Days and Became a Viral Media Sensation* (Phoenix: Instinct Media, 2014), 10.

143 *Cisna had quit his job as a high school teacher to become a paid McDonald's "brand ambassador"* Scott Stump, "Parents Protest 'McDonald's Diet' Ambassador for Speaking in Schools," *Today*, November 3, 2015, https://www.today.com/health/parents-protest-mcdonalds-diet-ambassador-speaking-schools-t53696.

144 *a quote which he misattributed to Mark Twain* 540 *Meals: Choices Make the Difference*; Center for Mark Twain Studies, "The Apocryphal Mark Twain: If You Don't Read the Newspaper, You're Uninformed. If You Do, You're Misinformed," February 21, 2018, http://marktwainstudies.com/the-apocryphal-twain-if-you-dont-read-the-newspaper-youre-uninformed-if-you-do-youre-misinformed/.

145   *I wrote a lengthy blog post about* **540 Meals** Bettina Elias Siegel,
      "'540 Meals': A McDonald's Infomercial Coming to a School
      Near You," *The Lunch Tray*, October 12, 2015, https://www
      .thelunchtray.com/cisna-540-meals-a-mcdonalds-infomercial-
      coming-to-a-school-near-you/.

145   *pieces about Cisna and the film had appeared in major news
      outlets* Bettina Elias Siegel, "McDonald's Pulls '540 Meals' From
      Internet Under Growing Barrage of Media Criticism," *The
      Lunch Tray*, October 14, 2015, http://www.thelunchtray.com/
      mcdonalds-pulls-540-meals-from-internet-under-growing-
      barrage-of-media-criticism/.

145   *[McDonald's] seemed eager to double down* Lisa Baertlein, "Iowa
      Teacher Takes His 'McDonald's Diet' to Schools, Irking Critics,"
      *Reuters*, October 14, 2015, https://www.reuters.com/article/us-
      mcdonalds-cisna/iowa-teacher-takes-his-mcdonalds-diet-to-
      schools-irking-critics-idUSKCN0S82WG20151014; Aimee
      Picchi, "Is a Teacher's 'McDonald's Diet' Education—or
      Marketing?" *CBS News*, October 16, 2015, http://www.cbsnews.
      com/news/is-a-teachers-mcdonalds-diet-education-or-
      marketing/.

146   *the story quoted me, linked to my initial blog post* Roberto A. Ferdman,
      "The Controversial Thing Kids Are Being Taught about McDonald's
      at School," *Washington Post*, October 29, 2015, https://www.
      washingtonpost.com/news/wonkblog/wp/2015/10/29/how-
      mcdonalds-is-using-schools-to-try-to-change-what-kids-eat/.
      This story ran under the print headline "How McDonald's Is Using
      Schools to Try to Change What Kids Eat."

146   *I was later contacted by producers from both* **Today** *and* **The
      Doctors** Bettina Elias Siegel, "My Appearance Re: McDonald's
      '540 Meals' on the Doctors Talk Show!" *The Lunch Tray*,
      December 17, 2015; Bettina Elias Siegel, "My Appearance on the
      Today Show Re: McDonald's '540 Meals,'" *The Lunch Tray*,
      November 3, 2015, https://www.thelunchtray.com/my-
      appearance-on-the-today-show-re-mcdonalds-540-meals/.

147   *the company told the* **Post** *that it had pulled the plug on the entire
      Cisna/540 Meals program* Roberto A. Ferdman, "McDonald's

Quietly Ended Controversial Program That Was Making Parents and Teachers Uncomfortable," *Washington Post*, May 13, 2016, https://www.washingtonpost.com/news/wonk/wp/2016/05/13/mcdonalds-is-no-longer-telling-kids-in-schools-that-eating-french-fries-most-days-is-fine/?utm_term=.15da60765b8d.

148 *"They'll start to look out of step"* Sarah Knapton, "Waitrose to Ban Sales of High-Caffeine Energy Drinks to Children Under 16," *Telegraph*, January 4, 2018, https://www.telegraph.co.uk/news/2018/01/04/waitrose-ban-sales-high-caffeine-energy-drinks-children-16/; Rebecca Smithers, "UK Supermarkets Ban Sales of Energy Drinks to Under-16s," *Guardian*, March 5, 2018, https://www.theguardian.com/lifeandstyle/2018/mar/05/uk-supermarkets-ban-sales-energy-drinks-under 16s.

149 *study has found that Brighter Bites actually does improve families' eating habits* Shreela V. Sharma et al., "Evaluating a School-Based Fruit and Vegetable Co-op in Low-Income Children: A Quasi-Experimental Study," *Preventive Medicine* 91 (2016): 8–17, doi:10.1016/j.ypmed.2016.07.022; Bettina Elias Siegel, "This Texas Nonprofit Is Helping Low-Income Families Eat More Fruits and Vegetables," *Civil Eats*, December 3, 2016, https://civileats.com/2016/07/18/how-a-texas-nonprofit-is-bringing-fresh-produce-to-low-income-families/; Brighter Bites website, www.brighterbites.org.

151 *1 parent = A fruitcake* I first came across "1 parent = a fruitcake" in promotional material created by Parents for Public Schools Houston, but the text seems to be generally popular in public school reform circles and I've been unable to track down the original source.

154 *there's now expert guidance on how much added sugar is too much for kids* Miriam B. Vos, "Added Sugars and Cardiovascular Disease Risk in Children: A Scientific Statement From the American Heart Association," *Circulation* 135, no. 19 (May 9, 2017): e1017–e1034, doi:10.1161/CIR.0000000000000439.

159 *a group called Healthy School Food Maryland* Donna St. George, "Report Card on School Food in Maryland: Lots of C's, One A,

Two B's," *Washington Post*, January 15, 2017, https://www.
washingtonpost.com/local/education/report-card-on-school-
food-in-maryland-lots-of-cs-one-a-two-bs/2017/01/15/
6a9bdf6a-d420-11e6-9cb0-54ab630851e8_story.html?utm_te
rm=.05a885e8dcda&noredirect=on.

## 9. Four Wishes

163 *the Minneapolis Healthy Corner Store initiative* Minneapolis
Health Department, "Healthy Corner Stores," http://www.
minneapolismn.gov/health/living/new%20cornerstores.

163 *The most effective measure…would be banning such child-
directed marketing* Sarah Boseley, "Obesity Experts Call for
Stricter Rules on Junk Food Ads Targeted at Children,"
*Guardian*, February 18, 2015, www.theguardian.com/society/
2015/feb/18/children-obesity-who-marketing-unhealthy-
food.

164 *such a ban is "an urgently needed strategy"* Harvard T. H. Chan
School of Public Health, "Food Marketing and Labeling," www.
hsph.harvard.edu/obesity-prevention-source/obesity-
prevention/food-environment/food-marketing-and-labeling-
and-obesity-prevention/; World Health Organization, "Set of
Recommendations on the Marketing of Foods and Non-
Alcoholic Beverages to Children," 2010, https://www.who.int/
dietphysicalactivity/publications/recsmarketing/en/;
Amandine Garde, Seamus Byrne, Nikhil Gokani, and Ben
Murphy, "A Child Rights-Based Approach to Food Marketing:
A Guide For Policy Makers," UNICEF report, April 20, 2018,
https://www.unicef.org/csr/files/A_Child_Rights-Based_
Approach_to_Food_Marketing_Report.pdf. For a discussion
of First Amendment concerns associated with such a ban,
see Samantha Graff, Dale Kunkel, and Seth E. Mermin,
"Government Can Regulate Food Advertising To Children
Because Cognitive Research Shows That It Is Inherently
Misleading," *Health Affairs* 31, no. 2 (2012): 392–98, doi:10.1377/
hlthaff.2011.0609.

164 *condemning all advertising to younger children because it unfairly exploits them* American Psychological Association, *Report of the APA Task Force on Advertising and Children,* February 20, 2004, www.apa.org/pi/families/resources/ advertising-children.pdf; "Perspectives on Marketing, Self-Regulation and Childhood Obesity," Federal Trade Commission Workshop remarks by Donald Shifrin, AAP Committee on Communications, July 14–15, 2005, Washington, DC, https:// www.aap.org/en-us/advocacy-and-policy/federal-advocacy/ Pages/Perspectives-on-Marketing,-Self-Regulation-and-Childhood-Obesity.aspx.

164 *Chile's government managed to overcome a decade of stiff industry opposition* Andrew Jacobs, "In Sweeping War on Obesity, Chile Slays Tony the Tiger," *New York Times,* February 7, 2018, www.nytimes.com/2018/02/07/health/obesity-chile-sugar-regulations.html.

164 *other countries … have long banned all advertising to children* The World Cancer Research Fund International, a nonprofit organization in the UK, maintains an active database of countries with restrictions on child-directed food and beverage advertising. It may be accessed at https://wcrf.org/sites/default/ files/Restrict-advertising.pdf.

164 *Seventy percent supported restricting unhealthy food and drink marketing* Jennifer L. Harris, Karen S. Haraghey, Yoon-Young Choi, and Frances Fleming-Milici, "Parents' Attitudes About Food Marketing to Children—2012 to 2015: Opportunities and Challenges to Creating Demand for a Healthier Food Environment," report from the UConn Rudd Center for Food Policy & Obesity, 2015, http://www.uconnruddcenter.org/ files/Pdfs/Rudd%20Center%20Parent%20Attitudes%20 Report%202017.pdf.

165 *prevent 129,100 cases of childhood obesity by 2025* Steven L. Gortmaker et al., "Cost Effectiveness of Childhood Obesity Interventions," *American Journal of Preventative Medicine* 49, no. 1 (July 2015): 102–11, doi.org/10.1016/j. amepre.2015.03.032.

166 *When children played an advergame sponsored by the produce company Dole* Jennifer L. Harris, Sarah E. Speers, Marlene B. Schwartz, and Kelly D. Brownell, "US Food Company Branded Advergames on the Internet: Children's Exposure and Effects on Snack Consumption," *Journal of Children and Media* 6, no. 1 (2012): 51–68, doi:10.1080/17482 798.2011.633405.

166 *they scored points every time a Pac-Man character ate healthy snacks* Tiffany A. Pempek and Sandra L. Calvert, "Tipping the Balance," *Archives of Pediatrics & Adolescent Medicine* 163, no. 7 (2009): 633, doi:10.1001/archpediatrics.2009.71.

166 *a deal brokered in 2013 by Michelle Obama's Partnership for a Healthier America* Helena Bottemiller Evich, "How the Produce Industry Got Elmo," *POLITICO*, November 4, 2013, https:// www.politico.com/story/2013/11/michelle-obama-sesame-street-obesity-099328.

166 *"Team FNV," a slick marketing campaign aimed at older children and adults* Elizabeth Crawford, "Fruits & Veggies Take on Packaged Food with FNV Ad Campaign Endorsed by the First Lady and Celebrities," *Food Navigator*, March 2, 2015, https:// www.foodnavigator-usa.com/Article/2015/03/02/Fruits-veggies-FNV-ad-campaign-endorsed-by-FLOTUS-and-celebrities.

166 *Seventy-nine percent of parents in the Rudd survey* Harris, Haraghey, Choi, and Fleming-Milici, "Parents' Attitudes About Food Marketing to Children."

167 *"If you're not hungry enough to eat an apple, then you're probably not hungry"* Michael Pollan, *Food Rules: An Eater's Manual* (New York: Penguin Books, 2009), 105.

167 *58 percent admitted "most days I probably should be eating healthier"* Cary Funk and Brian Kennedy, "The New Food Fights: U.S. Public Divides Over Food Science," Pew Research Center: Internet, Science & Technology, December 1, 2016, http://www.pewinternet.org/2016/12/01/the-new-food-fights/.

168 *the University of Minnesota's School of Public Health followed more than 1,100 young adults* Jennifer Utter et al., "Self-Perceived

Cooking Skills in Emerging Adulthood Predict Better Dietary Behaviors and Intake 10 Years Later: A Longitudinal Study," *Journal of Nutrition Education and Behavior* 50, no. 5 (2018): 494–500. doi:10.1016/j.jneb.2018.01.021.

168 *In 2014, the Charlie Cart Project held a successful Kickstarter campaign* The Charlie Cart Project website, www.charliecart .org.

169 *a 2017 study by the Tisch Food Center at Teachers College, Columbia University* FoodCorps website, www.foodcorps.org; Pam Koch et al., "FoodCorps: Creating Healthy School Environments," Laurie M. Tisch Center for Food, Education & Policy, Program in Nutrition, Teachers College, Columbia University, February 2017, https://foodcorps.org/cms/assets/ uploads/2016/06/FoodCorps-Creating-Healthy-School-Environments-Teachers-College.pdf.

169 *a 2018 study from the University of Eastern Finland* Kaisa Kähkönen et al., "Sensory-Based Food Education in Early Childhood Education and Care, Willingness to Choose and Eat Fruit and Vegetables, and the Moderating Role of Maternal Education and Food Neophobia," *Public Health Nutrition* 21, no. 13 (September 2018): 2443–53, doi:10.1017/ s1368980018001106; Taejung Woo and Kyung-Hea Lee, "Effects of Sensory Education Based on Classroom Activities for Lower Grade School Children," *Nutrition Research and Practice* 7, no. 4 (August 2013): 336–41, doi:10.4162/nrp. 2013.7.4.336.

170 *"We cast the executives behind food marketing as controlling adult authority figures"* Christopher J. Bryan et al., "Harnessing Adolescent Values to Motivate Healthier Eating," *Proceedings of the National Academy of Sciences* 113, no. 39 (2016): 10830–35, doi:10.1073/pnas.1604586113; Amanda Ripley, "Can Teenage Defiance Be Manipulated for Good?" *New York Times*, September 12, 2016, https://www.nytimes.com/2016/09/13/ upshot/can-teenage-defiance-be-manipulated-for-good. html?smid=tw-share.

171 *"you empower them to take a stand"* Ripley, "Teenage Defiance."

171 *"Mr. Zee's Apple Factory"* Mr. Zee's Apple Factory, https://www.youtube.com/watch?v=xEN4UTbovKM.

171 *"We believe that all of our food can be part of a balanced lifestyle"* BalanceUS.org. http://www.balanceus.org; Yum! Brands 2014 Corporate Social Responsibility Report, http://www.yumcsr.com/pdf/2014_CSR_Report_040115.pdf.

171 *In 2011, researchers at Johns Hopkins found* Sara N. Bleich, Bradley J. Herring, Desmond D. Flagg, and Tiffany L. Gary-Webb, "Reduction in Purchases of Sugar-Sweetened Beverages Among Low-Income Black Adolescents After Exposure to Caloric Information," *American Journal of Public Health* 102, no. 2 (2012): 329–35, doi:10.2105/ajph.2011.300350.

172 *the improvement in kids' buying habits persisted...even after the signs were taken down* Sara N. Bleich, Colleen L. Barry, Tiffany L. Gary-Webb, and Bradley J. Herring, "Reducing Sugar-Sweetened Beverage Consumption by Providing Caloric Information: How Black Adolescents Alter Their Purchases and Whether the Effects Persist," *American Journal of Public Health* 104, no. 12 (2014): 2417–24, doi:10.2105/ajph.2014.302150.

172 *82 percent said they'd felt "tricked" by nutrition labeling* Zoya Gervis, "Most People Think Food Labels Are Misleading," *New York Post*, June 7, 2018, https://nypost.com/2018/06/07/most-people-think-food-labels-are-misleading/.

172 *In another recent poll, 52 percent of low-income parents* C.S. Mott Children's Hospital, National Poll on Children's Health, "Healthy Eating for Children: Parents Not Following the Recipe," February 20, 2017, https://mottpoll.org/reports-surveys/healthy-eating-children-parents-not-following-recipe.

172 *a simple front-of-package coding system* Marion Nestle, "IOM Releases Tough Report on Front-of-Package Labeling," *Food Politics*, October 20, 2011, https://www.foodpolitics.com/2011/10/iom-releases-tough-report-on-front-of-package-labeling/. (Nestle presciently noted when the IOM released its front-of-package proposal, "I'm guessing that anything this clear and understandable will elicit storms of protest.")

173 *"Wondering what all those numbers are?"* Facts Up Front
website, www.factsupfront.org.

173 *almost 44 percent of Chileans surveyed said they were paying
attention to the symbols* Ministry of Health, Chile (MINSAL),
"Informe De Evaluación De La Implementación De La Ley
Sobre Composición Nutricional De Los Alimentos Y Su
Publicidad," June 2017, https://www.minsal.cl/wp-content/
uploads/2017/05/Informe-Implementaci%C3%B3n-Ley-
20606-junio-2017-PDF.pdf.

173 *"Free of Logos [referring to the stop signs], Equally Rich"* Jacobs,
"Chile Slays Tony the Tiger"; Deborah A. Cohen, "Why Chile
Should Continue Placing 'Stop Signs' on Unhealthy Foods,"
RAND Corporation, March 19, 2018, https://www.rand.org/
blog/2018/03/fighting-obesity-why-chile-should-continue-
placing-stop.html.

173 *early data from Ecuador indicates that the color coding is indeed
encouraging shoppers* Rebecca Kanter, Lana Vanderlee, and
Stefanie Vandevijvere, "Front-of-Package Nutrition Labeling
Policy: Global Progress and Future Directions," *Public Health
Nutrition* 21, no. 8 (2018): 1399–408, doi:10.1017/
s1368980018000010.

175 *one school even saw a 40 percent drop in nurse's visits* Action
for Healthy Kids, "Recess Before Lunch," http://www
.actionforhealthykids.org/tools-for-schools/find-challenges/
cafeteria-challenges/1232-recess-before-lunch; Tara Parker-
Pope, "Seeing Benefits in Moving Recess Ahead of Lunch at
School," *New York Times*, January 26, 2010, https://www
.nytimes.com/2010/01/26/health/26well.html?mtrref=www
.google.com; "Timing and Duration Matters for School Lunch
and Recess," *Science Daily*, April 24, 2017, https://www
.sciencedaily.com/releases/2017/04/170424084025.htm.

176 *too-short lunch periods also deprive kids of the chance to learn*
Maria Godoy and Allison Aubrey, "Kids Who Are Time-
Crunched at School Lunch Toss More and Eat Less," *NPR*,
September 24, 2015, https://www.npr.org/sections/thesalt/

2015/09/24/439487395/kids-who-are-time-crunched-at-school-lunch-toss-more-and-eat-less.

177 *a marketing organization created by the USDA* Michael Moss, "While Warning About Fat, U.S. Pushes Cheese Sales," *New York Times*, November 6, 2010, https://www.nytimes.com/2010/11/07/us/07fat.html.

178 *each slice [of Domino's Smart Slice] contains two ounces of cheese* Judy Hall, "Why the Dairy Checkoff Partnered with Domino's," *Progressive Dairyman*, May 6, 2016, https://www.progressivedairy.com/news/organizations/why-the-dairy-checkoff-partnered-with-domino-s; My Plate nutrition education for teens accessed at https://www.choosemyplate.gov/ten-tips-choose-the-foods-you-need-to-grow; Moss, "While Warning About Fat, U.S. Pushes Cheese Sales."

178 *"we want to make sure there's always an outlet for it"* Domino's promotional Smart Slice video accessed at https://www.youtube.com/watch?v=IXFHbabmlFI.

178 *But the dairy industry . . . successfully lobbied President Trump's USDA in 2018 to ignore that advice* Peter Robinson and Lydia Mulvany, "Big Dairy Is About to Flood America's School Lunches with Milk," *Bloomberg*, January 9, 2019, https://www.bloomberg.com/news/features/2019-01-09/big-dairy-is-about-to-flood-america-s-school-lunches-with-milk.

178 *This arrangement dates back to the beginning of the National School Lunch Program* Janet Poppendieck, *Free for All: Fixing School Food in America* (Berkeley: University of California Press, 2010), 48-49.

180 *In France, for example, school meal prices are tied to family income* Bettina Elias Siegel, "The Real Problem With Lunch," *New York Times*, January 16, 2016, https://www.nytimes.com/2016/01/16/opinion/the-real-problem-with-lunch.html; Chico Harlan, "On Japan's School Lunch Menu: A Healthy Meal, Made from Scratch," *Washington Post*, January 26, 2013, https://www.washingtonpost.com/world/on-japans-school-lunch-menu-a-healthy-meal-made-from-scratch/2013/01/26/5f31d208-63a2-11e2-85f5-a8a9228e55e7_story.

html?noredirect=on&utm_term=.7f2c355f4ca8; Karen Le Billon, "French School Lunch Menus," *KarenLeBillon.com*, March 18, 2012, https://karenlebillon.com/french-school-lunch-menus/.

181 *a nationwide deficit estimated to be $5 billion in 2014* Bettina Elias Siegel, "In the Case of School Lunch, Kitchens Might Be as Important as Ingredients," *Civil Eats*, April 14, 2016, https://civileats.com/2016/02/16/in-the-case-of-school-lunch-kitchens-might-be-as-important-as-ingredients/.

182 *Janet Poppendieck pegged the additional cost at $12 billion as of 2009* Poppendieck, *Free for All*, 257–296.

## 10. We're Better Than This

184 *Miller...proclaimed that his first official act would be "declaring amnesty" for cupcakes* Eva Hershaw, "Agriculture Commissioner Grants Amnesty to Cupcakes in First Official Act," *Texas Tribune*, January 13, 2015, https://www.texastribune.org/2015/01/12/commissioner-sid-miller-gives-amnesty-cupcakes/.

185 *Texas has had a state law on its books since 2005* Bettina Elias Siegel, "'Cupcake Amnesty': Childhood Obesity and the Political Divide," *The Lunch Tray*, January 12, 2015, https://www.thelunchtray.com/cupcake-amnesty-childhood-obesity-political-divide/; Eva Hershaw, "Commissioner Gets Cupcake Policy Wrong, Combs Says," *Texas Tribune*, January 14, 2015, https://www.texastribune.org/2015/01/14/cupcakes-legal-texas-schools-ten-years/.

185 *This so-called Safe Cupcake Amendment also supersedes any local policies* Siegel, "Cupcake Amnesty."

185 *Miller['s]...seemingly brash policies...were widely reported in local and national media* Bettina Elias Siegel, "Ag Commissioner Miller on Fox News: Distortions as Big as the State of Texas," *The Lunch Tray*, January 20, 2015, https://www.thelunchtray.com/ag-commissioner-miller-fox-news-distortions-big-state-texas/; Ian Tuttle, "TX to Grant Massive Amnesty—to

Classroom Cupcakes," *National Review*, October 10, 2017, https://www.nationalreview.com/corner/tx-grant-massive-amnesty-classroom-cupcakes-ian-tuttle/.

185 *when Miller did reverse the (diet) soda and (obsolete) fryer bans* Nathan Koppel, "Texas Agriculture Chief: Don't Mess With Our Deep-Fried Food," *Wall Street Journal*, April 27, 2015, https://www.wsj.com/articles/texas-agriculture-chief-dont-mess-with-our-deep-fried-food-1430178526; Kate McGee, "Fried Food in School Cafeterias: 'It's About Freedom and Liberty,' Says Ag Commissioner," *KUT*, April 20, 2015, http://www.kut.org/post/fried-food-school-cafeterias-its-about-freedom-and-liberty-says-ag-commissioner.

186 *he later made the short list to head up President Trump's Department of Agriculture* Helena Bottemiller Evich and Ian Kullgren, "Cupcake Defender Interviews for Ag Secretary Job," *POLITICO*, December 30, 2016, https://www.politico.com/story/2016/12/sid-miller-agriculture-commissioner-cupcakes-vegetables-233069.

186 *[Miller's] website currently makes the absurd claim* "Healthy Kids Not Healthy Trashcans," www.millerfortexas.com.

186 *a vocal champion of getting more fresh, local produce into schools, and his office awards generous grants* Bottemiller Evich and Kullgren, "Cupcake Defender Interviews for Ag Secretary Job"; nutrition education grant information accessed on the Texas Department of Agriculture website, http://www.texasagriculture.gov/GrantsServices/TradeandBusinessDevelopment/3EsGrantPrograms/Establishing3Es.aspx.

186 *five years earlier, he'd warmly praised those same efforts* Kylie Atwood, "Chris Christie: Keep the White House Out of the Cafeteria," *CBS News*, January 18, 2016, https://www.cbsnews.com/news/chris-christie-keep-the-white-house-out-of-the-cafeteria/ (quoting "Michelle Obama Gets a Republican Boost on Obesity Campaign," *Telegraph*, February 28, 2011, https://www.telegraph.co.uk/news/worldnews/northamerica/usa/8351299/Michelle-Obama-gets-a-Republican-boost-on-obesity-campaign.html?sms_ss=facebook&at_xt=4d6b600367b25fe3,0).

186  *"leave us alone, get off our back"* Sam Stein, "Palin Slams Michelle Obama Again, This Time for Anti-Obesity Campaign," *Huffington Post*, November 24, 2010, https://www.huffingtonpost.com/2010/11/24/palin-slams-michelle-obam_n_788200.html.

186  *Palin had asked for more state funding to combat childhood obesity* Eric Boehlert, "Nanny State Alert: Gov. Palin Urged 'Healthy Habits in Eating' for Alaskans," *Media Matters for America*, February 23, 2011, https://www.mediamatters.org/blog/2011/02/23/nanny-state-alert-gov-palin-urged-healthy-habit/176767.

186  *a period of particularly intense food tribalism in this country* Cary Funk and Brian Kennedy, "The New Food Fights: U.S. Public Divides Over Food Science," Pew Research Center: Internet, Science & Technology, December 1, 2016, http://www.pewinternet.org/2016/12/01/the-new-food-fights/.

187  *William Henry Harrison, was the everyman living on "raw beef and salt"* Harvey A. Levenstein, *Revolution at the Table: The Transformation of the American Diet* (Berkeley: University of California Press, 2003), 10–11.

187  *Barack Obama asked for Grey Poupon* Dahlia Lithwick, "The Dreaded Broccoli Uprising and Other Nutty GOP Nightmares," *Slate*, December 21, 2010, https://slate.com/news-and-politics/2010/12/the-dreaded-broccoli-uprising-and-other-nutty-gop-nightmares.html; Jake Miller, "Five Times Politicians Failed at Food," *CBS News*, April 8, 2015, https://www.cbsnews.com/news/five-times-politicians-failed-at-food/.

187  *feel compelled to eat lots of fried-things-on-a-stick* Maxwell Tani, "Here Are the Best Pictures of the Presidential Candidates Eating Greasy, Fried Food at Iowa State Fair," *Connecticut Post*, August 19, 2015, https://www.ctpost.com/technology/businessinsider/article/Here-s-all-the-greasy-fatty-fried-food-6446286.php.

187  *"Somebody get a f---ing corn dog in his hand—now!"* Amy Chozick, "Too Fit to Be President?" *Wall Street Journal*, August 2, 2008, https://www.wsj.com/articles/SB121755336096303089.

187   the "Diabetes Belt"—a swath of Southern and Southeastern states Centers for Disease Control and Prevention, "CDC Identifies Diabetes Belt," https://www.cdc.gov/diabetes/pdfs/data/diabetesbelt.pdf; Paul Krugman, "Heavy Politics," New York Times, March 5, 2015, https://krugman.blogs.nytimes.com/2015/03/05/heavy-politics/.

188   attacks that... Meghan Daum described... as... "astonishingly ugly" Meghan Daum, "A Feeding Frenzy," Los Angeles Times, March 3, 2011, http://articles.latimes.com/2011/mar/03/opinion/la-oe-daum-michelle-20110303.

188   historically directing less than 10 percent of their political contributions Vince Dixon, "Interactive: How Much Are Restaurant Chains Donating to Republicans and Democrats?" Eater, February 8, 2016, https://www.eater.com/2016/2/8/10904984/restaurant-PACS-political-donations; "Restaurants & Drinking Establishments," OpenSecrets.org, https://www.opensecrets.org/industries/indus.php?ind=G2900l; "Food Processing & Sales," OpenSecrets.org, http://www.opensecrets.org/industries/indus.php?ind=A09; Duff Wilson and Janet Roberts, "Special Report: How Washington Went Soft on Childhood Obesity," Reuters, April 27, 2012, https://www.reuters.com/article/us-usa-foodlobby/special-report-how-washington-went-soft-on-childhood-obesity-idUSBRE83Q0ED20120427.

189   clearer product labeling "eat[s] away at consumer freedoms" Ashe Schow, "First Lady Michelle Obama Thinks You're Too Dumb to Read a Nutrition Label," Washington Examiner, February 27, 2014, https://www.washingtonexaminer.com/first-lady-michelle-obama-thinks-youre-too-dumb-to-read-a-nutrition-label; Daniel J. Popeo, "Food Labeling and the Nanny State," Forbes, April 25, 2013, https://www.forbes.com/sites/docket/2011/06/30/food-labeling-and-the-nanny-state/#7acf08e35ded.

189   these critics often make a case for free-market solutions Popeo, "Food Labeling and the Nanny State."

189   ten... corporations... control almost every major food and beverage brand we buy Kate Taylor, "These 10 Companies

Control Everything You Buy," *Business Insider*, April 4, 2017, https://www.businessinsider.com/10-companies-control-food-industry-2017-3.

189 *"she cannot trust parents to make decisions for their own children"* Stein, "Palin Slams Michelle Obama Again."

191 *an astonishing 72 percent increase in medical evacuations* Mission: Readiness, Council for a Strong America, "Unhealthy and Unprepared," October 2018, https://www.strongnation.org/articles/737-unhealthy-and-unprepared.

192 *annual medical spending due to obesity was nearly $150 billion* Beth Baker, "Obesity's Hefty Price Tag," *POLITICO*, March 8, 2017, https://www.politico.com/agenda/story/2017/03/obesity-epidemic-in-america-healthcare-costs-000336.

192 *"the two parties might find a way to cooperate"* David S. Ludwig, *Always Hungry?: Conquer Cravings, Retrain Your Fat Cells, and Lose Weight Permanently* (New York: Grand Central Life & Style, 2016), 32.

192 *The Grocery Manufacturers Association...recently saw its membership dwindle* Helena Bottemiller Evich and Catherine Boudreau, "The Big Washington Food Fight," *POLITICO*, November 26, 2017, https://www.politico.com/story/2017/11/26/food-lobby-consumer-tastes-washington-190528.

192 *the Rudd Center for Food Policy & Obesity's 2015 parent survey* Jennifer L. Harris, Karen S. Haraghey, Yoon-Young Choi, and Frances Fleming-Milici, "Parents' Attitudes About Food Marketing to Children: 2012 to 2015: Opportunities and Challenges to Creating Demand for a Healthier Food Environment," report from the UConn Rudd Center for Food Policy & Obesity, April 2017, http://www.uconnruddcenter.org/files/Pdfs/Rudd%20Center%20Parent%20Attitudes%20Report%202017.pdf.

193 *African American and Hispanic parents may be even more willing to engage on these issues* Harris, Haraghey, Choi, and Fleming-Milici, "Parents' Attitudes About Food Marketing to Children: 2012 to 2015."

# INDEX

Note: Page references followed by an "*f*" indicate figures.

Children's Food and Beverage Advertising
Initiative (CFBAI) (continued)
"healthier dietary choices," definition of,
83, 87
history of, 82–83
IWG and, 85–88
licensed characters and, 84
loopholes in pledge, 83–84, 88
Michelle Obama and, 85–86
nutrition standards, 87
pledge, 83–84
product packaging and, 84
schools, marketing in, 84
Sensible Food Policy Coalition and,
85–86
children's menus
calories and, 29, 130–31
candy on, 20, 28
children's behavior and, 130
Chili's, 20–21, 28
Friendly's, 20–21, 28
history of, 15–21
improvements to, 27–29, 130, 192
Kids LiveWell initiative, 27–29
Michelle Obama and, 27–28
picky eating and, 6–7, 20–21
portion sizes, 130–31
pricing, 129–30
Red Robin, 20, 28
Silver Diner, 28
sugary beverages and, 20–21, 28, 130
Chile, food marketing reforms, 164, 173
Chili's, 20–21, 28
Choicelunch, 104, 177
Christie, Chris, 13, 186
Cisna, John, 142–47
classroom. See school classroom
"clean label" foods, 7, 31
Coalition of Sustainable School Meal
Programs, 97
Coca Cola
contributions to health organizations, 63
Global Energy Balance Network, 63
market power, 189

product reformulation in Chile, 173
sponsorship of dietitians, 64
Colson, Ethel Maude, 16–18, 19, 21, 28–29
commercials, television. See marketing to
children; marketing to parents
commodities. See agricultural commodities,
in school food
Common Sense Book of Baby and Child Care,
26–27
competitive food, 105–6
ConAgra
Kid Cuisine relaunch, 66–68
school food commodity processing, 104
sponsorship of School Nutrition
Association, 97
confusion, about nutrition
front groups and, 64
industry-sown, 61–66
among parents, 56, 61, 67, 128
among registered dietitians, 61
solutions to address, 172–74
Cooke, Lucy, 32, 38, 40, 45, 46–47
cookies
in babies' and toddlers' diets, 126–27
as "kid food" grocery category, 23, 127–28
Girl Scout Mango Creme, 55
in school breakfast, 4–5
as ultra-processed food, x
cooking. See also home economics
decline in, 21, 42–44
at home, 9, 21, 42–43
from scratch, in school meals, 4, 103, 104,
107, 149
short-order, and picky eating, 32, 33,
skills, effect on diet, 168
socioeconomics and, 42–43
teaching children to, 138, 168
Cooper, Anderson, 141
Cooper, Ann, 101, 105, 106, 107, 108, 178,
179, 180, 181, 182
"copycat" foods and beverages, 92–93,
95–98. See also à la carte foods and
beverages
defense of, 98

Hauser, Gayelord, 8
"health halo" marketing, 52–57
healthcare costs, obesity related, 164,
191–92
"healthy," definition of, 53, 61, 65
Healthy, Hunger-Free Kids Act
(HHFKA). See also school food
competitive food and, 105–6
"copycat" foods and beverages and, 93,
95–96
food waste and, 94
improvement of school meals,
93–94, 174
"Letter of the Law" school meals and,
96–98
Michelle Obama and, 93, 188
restrictive regulations of, 179
school fundraisers and, 110–12
Smart Snacks regulations, 105–6,
110–12, 175, 187
sugar and, 95
wellness policies and, 155
healthy food, kids embracing, 167–72
heart disease, 135
Helfman, Lisa, 148
HHFKA. See Healthy, Hunger–Free
Kids Act
high fructose corn syrup, 66
highly processed food
in children's diets, 124–25
cost of, 33
definition of, x–xii
effect on family dinner, 43–44
health concerns associated with, xii,
133–35
as "kid food," 2, 116–17
Mommy Wars and, 12
nutrition claims for, 52–54
phytochemicals and, 126
picky eating and, 31, 35–36, 96
satiety and, 126
in school meals, 4, 96, 104, 105, 133,
174, 176, 178, 180
socioeconomic status and, 37

HISD. See Houston Independent School
District
home economics, 17, 43, 168
House Agriculture Committee, 99
Houston Independent School District
(HISD), 2–5, 102, 111–12, 151,
157–58, 160
hunger cues, 41, 59, 121, 133–34, 166

In Defense of Mothers: How to Bring Up
Children in Spite of the More Zealous
Psychologists, 26
infants. See baby and toddler foods; babies
and toddlers, diet of
"information laundering," 64
"inoculation," against food and beverage
marketing, 170–72
Instagram, 65. See also social media
Institute of Medicine (IOM), 82–83, 97,
172, 178, 188
Interagency Working Group on Food
Marketed to Children (IWG), 85–88.
See also CFBAI; marketing to children
International Food Information Council, 64
International Life Sciences Institute, 64
IOM. See Institute of Medicine
IWG. See Interagency Working Group on
Food Marketed to Children

Jacobson, Lisa, 70
Jarrett, Valerie, 86
Johns Hopkins, 79, 171
joint pain, 135
juice. See also sugary beverages
in Afterschool Snack Program, 117
"baby juice," 129
in Child and Adult Care Food
Program, 117
children's consumption of, 22, 23,
128–29
children's menus and, 129
"health halo" of, 61, 128–29
recommended quota for children, 129
in school meals, 95, 129

standardized testing and, 5, 109–10, 115, 120
sugar in, 128
in WIC, 129
junk food. See highly processed food

Kanner, Leo, 26
Katz, David, 138, 139
Kellogg's, 51, 76, 86, 97, 102, 175–76, 189
Kerry, John, 187
KFC, 51
Kid Cuisine, 66–68
"kid food"
  breakfast cereal as, 23
  characteristics of, 22–24
  children's taste preferences, effect on, 27, 31, 37
  children's view of, 23
  Clara Davis studies and, 27, 29
  definition of, 22–23, 27
  "fun" and, 23
  grocery products, 23, 127
  parent survey about, 22–24
  sugar and, 23, 127–28
  ubiquity of, 23–24, 27–29
Kidfresh, 56
"Kid/Mom Dynamic," 66–68, 66f
Kids LiveWell initiative, 27–29
Kid Vid, 81–82, 85, 87
Klobuchar, Amy, 97
Kraft Heinz, 51, 84, 97, 104
Kuzemchak, Sally, 154, 157–58

labels. See product packaging and labeling
Lappé, Frances Moore, 8
lean, finely textured beef (LFTB), 141.
  See also "pink slime"
Leo Burnett, 60
Let's Move! initiative, 85–86, 108
LFTB. See lean, finely textured beef
licensed characters, 74, 83–84
liver. See nonalcoholic fatty liver disease (NAFLD)
Living Loud, 49

local school wellness policies. See wellness policies
"lookalike" foods and beverages.
  See "copycat" foods and beverages
Ludwig, David, 133–34, 192
lunch, school. See school food
"lunch shaming," 10, 182
The Lunch Tray blog, 9, 32, 114–15, 140–41
  Food-in-the-Classroom Manifesto, 120–22

MacDougall, Alice Foote, 18–19
Mak, Veronica Sau-Wa, 60
marketing, food and beverage industry.
  See marketing to children; marketing to parents; marketing to schools marketing to children. See also CFBAI; Pester Power
  ban on, 163–67
  cartoon characters and, 74–75
  celebrities and, 75–76
  childhood obesity and, 79, 82–83
  children of color and, 79, 193
  developmental psychology and, 73–74, 80
  digital, 76–77
  expenditures on, 72–73
  540 Meals, 142–47
  harms of, 78–80
  of healthy foods, 165–66
  industry self-regulation and, 82–89
  Kid Cuisine, 67–68
  Kid Vid and, 81–82, 85, 87
  licensed characters and, 74, 83–84
  Michelle Obama and, 85–86
  parents' views about, 80, 164–65, 192–93
  "priming" and, 79
  product placements, 78, 80
  rise of, 70–71
  in schools, 78, 84, 142–47
  social media and, 76–77, 80
  sports figures and, 75–76
  "surround marketing," 77–78
  tax code, use of, to curb, 165
  team sports and, 78

marketing to children (*continued*)
on television, 70, 76, 77–78, 81, 84, 88, 192
undermining parents through, 78–81
marketing to parents, 48–68
confusion about nutrition, industry-sown, 61–66, 67
"dietitian approved" claims, 64–66
front-of-package nutrition ratings, 172–73
"fruitwashing," 52–53, 173–74
"health-halo" techniques, 52–57, 173–74
"healthwashing," 52–57, 173–74
Kid Cuisine, 66–68
"Kid/Mom Dynamic," 66–68, 66*f*
"made with" claims, 2, 52–53, 173–74
nutrient claims, 52–54, 173–74
nutrition shakes and, 59–60
"peace and quiet" appeals, 51–52, 129–30
"pediatrician recommended" claims, 58
picky-eating appeals, 50–51, 58–60
toddler milks and, 57–59
"veggie-sneaking" and, 54–57, 173–74
marketing to schools, 84, 97–98, 100, 102
Mars, Inc., 148, 189
Marshall Fields, 19–20
McDonalds
chicken nugget, invention of, 20
children's menu, 130
dietitians, paid 64–65
*540 Meals*, 9, 142–47
LeBron James and, 75
marketing to children, 2, 78, 84
media literacy, teaching children, 138, 170-72
menus. *See* children's menus; school food
military, effect of obesity on, 191
milk. *See also* dairy industry; toddler milks
flavored, 3, 12, 92, 95, 133, 156, 178
historical child feeding advice and, 19
picky eating and, 35
in school meals, 178
Miller, Sid, 184–86

Minneapolis Healthy Corner Store initiative, 163
Mission: Readiness, 191
moderation. *See* "calorie-balancing" messaging
"mom bloggers," 65–66
Mondelez, 189
Monteiro, Carlos, x
mood, food and, 134–35
*Mother Jones*, 98
Mr. Potato Head, 70
"Mr. Zee's Apple Factory," 171
Muth, Natalie Digate, 58
*My McDonald's Diet*, 143
My Plate, 177

NAFLD. *See* nonalcoholic fatty liver disease
"The Nag Factor," 71
nagging. *See* Pester Power
"nanny state" messaging, 13, 81, 82, 183, 188–90
National Academy of Medicine, 82
National Confectioners Association, 62
National Dairy Council, 177
National Farm-to-School Network, 108
National Restaurant Association, 28
National School Lunch Program 4, 98–99, 154, 177, 178. *See also* Healthy, Hunger-Free Kids Act; school food
Nestlé, 86, 189
Nestle, Marion, 63
neuroscience, in marketing to children, 73–74
*New York Times*, 10, 63, 76, 141
nonalcoholic fatty liver disease (NAFLD), 132–33
NOVA classification system, x–xii
"nutrient standard" school menu planning, 5
nutrients
brain and, 134
discovery of, 17, 61
fortification of, 125

pediatricians (*continued*)
  historical feeding advice, 24–26
  Kid Vid and, 95
  PediaSure and, 60
  "recommended by" claims, 57–58
PepsiCo, 97, 189
Pertschuk, Michael, 81, 82
Pester Power. *See also* marketing to
    children
  industry acknowledgment of, 71
  Kid Cuisine and, 67
  potency of, 69–70, 72
  products which inspire most, 70
  rise of, 70–71
  undermining of parents, 79
petitions, 9, 141–42, 145–46, 147–48,
    150, 181, 192. *See also* Change.org;
    food advocacy
physical activity. *See also* "calorie-balancing"
    messaging
  Coca-Cola on, 63
  *540 Meals* on, 143–44
  Global Energy Balance Network on, 63
  Let's Move! initiative on, 86
  and obesity, 124
  and sports drinks, 115–16
phytochemicals, 126
picky eating, 30–47
  anxiety and shyness, role of, 35
  bitterness, children's aversion to, and,
    34–35
  breastfeeding and, 41
  children's menus and, 6–7, 20–21
  Division of Responsibility and, 42–47
  "flavor window" and, 39, 41
  food neophobia and, 34
  formula feeding and, 41
  genetics, role of, 35
  highly processed food and, 31, 37
  historical feeding advice, 45
  industry exploitation of, 47, 50–59
  innate causes, 34–36
  introduction of solid food and, 38–40
  nutrition shake marketing and, 59–60

as "pain point," 47
  parenting style and, 37–38, 45–47
  parents' frustration over, 32–33, 36
  parents' perception of, 36, 38
  prenatal diet and, 40–41
  pressure and, 37–38, 41
  rice cereal and, 38–39
  salt, children's attraction to, and, 36
  short-order cooking and, 32, 33
  snacking and, 44
  socioeconomic status and, 33, 37, 41
  sugar, children's attraction to, and
    35–36
  "super-tasters" and, 35
  toddler milk marketing and, 58
  toddler squeeze pouches and, 39–40,
    44–45
Pingree, Chellie, 142
"pink slime," 9. *See also* lean, finely
    textured beef
pizza
  childhood obesity and, 131
  children's consumption of, 126, 131
  on children's menus, 20
  as classroom reward, 113
  Domino's Smart Slice pizza, 93, 95, 100,
    102, 177–78
  as "kid food," 22
  OH YES! 56
  in school meals, 90, 91, 93, 97, 102,
    104, 106
Plum Organics, 40, 44, 56
politics, partisan, 13, 183, 185–89, 192
Pollan, Michael, xi, 53, 167
Poppendieck, Janet, 4, 91, 182
PopTropica, 6
portion size, on children's menus, 130–31
potatoes, 3, 5, 92, 97, 127, 174. *See also*
    French fries
poverty. *See* socioeconomic status;
    socioeconomic stigma
prenatal diet, 40–41
"priming," 79
processed food. *See* highly processed food